i

Geriatric Nursing Care Plans

WITHDRAWN

Marie S. Jaffe

Skidmore-Roth Publishing, Inc.

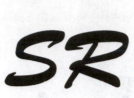

Skidmore-Roth

Editor: Linda Skidmore-Roth, R.N., M.S.N., N.P.
Cover design: Scott Mathews
Typesetting: Affiliated Executive Systems

Notice: The author(s) and the publisher of this volume have taken care to make certain that all information is correct and compatible with the standards generally accepted at the time of publication.

Skidmore-Roth Publishing, Inc.
2620 S. Parker Road, Suite 147
Aurora, Colorado 80014
800-825-3150

Introductory Remarks

An ever-increasing elderly population requires the necessity for all health care personnel to become aware of the special needs and problems of this group. The need for education and skills in the care of chronic illnesses and long term care management is essential in providing and maintaining the health and functional capabilities of aged clients. Care of the elderly may take place in the home, hospital, long term care facility, alternative care facility, retirement community and outpatient clinic. Regardless of the environment or type of practitioner who delivers the care, a sensitivity to aging and its values, capabilities and importance of dignity is important if one is to perform safe, meaningful care and assistance to this population.

Health care in the elderly creates the largest expenditure of a client's economic resources if a chronic illness or disability is present and often leads to poverty and/or deprivation in other human needs areas. This, in turn, affects prevention of complications or the development of additional health problems which further compromises the physical, psychosocial and economic needs of these individuals. The most common chronic illnesses of the elderly are heart conditions, chronic obstructive pulmonary diseases, hypertension, arthritis, and sensory deficits (visual, auditory). Pneumonia is the most common infectious disease necessitating hospitalization of the elderly. Seven chronic diseases accounts for 80% of deaths in the elderly; heart disease, malignant neoplasms, stroke, chronic obstructive pulmonary disease, atherosclerosis and kidney disease. Acute conditions such as pneumonia, influenza, accidents and adverse effects accidents and septicemia made up the balance of the ten leading causes of death in the elderly.

The fields of geriatrics which may be defined as care of the ill elderly and gerontology which may be defined as a science of the aging process are used in medicine and nursing today. This book of care plans focuses on physical and psychosocial problems that compromise the health of an elderly client and has adopted the geriatric label in its title.

The focus of the second edition has been revised and additions made to reflect the care of the client/resident in a long-term facility. It has retained its adaptation to care in other types of facilities and environments as well. Every aspect of each plan has been updated and revised to include new NANDA diagnoses and provide broader and more in-depth information. Care plans have been expanded to include a total of forty-two general titles, sixteen of which provide forty-one inclusions of related conditions. Ten to eleven general and sub-inclusion titles have been added to this edition. The two sections in the appendix have been revised to include six extensive informative divisions.

My appreciation and thanks again is extended to Linda Skidmore-Roth, and her staff member, Sheila Passin-Swall, for their assistance in the development of this second edition.

Marie S. Jaffe

Using the Geriatric Care Plans

These plans have been developed to reflect physical and functional titles listed according to body systems or psychosocial problems. Included are the most common problems associated with the aging adult. Each system includes an Overview of the general system, General physiological changes associated with the aging process and Essential nursing diagnoses and care plans that are usually identified with the particular system. These essential nursing diagnoses and care plans may be cross-referenced with plans for conditions within the system or with plans for conditions within other systems if they apply. Each essential nursing diagnosis and care plan developed for the system includes:

- Nursing diagnosis as stated in NANDA taxonomy

- All of the related factors or risk factors and the defining characteristics specific to each related factor that have a relationship with the conditions associated with the older adult that could be applicable to any system

- Outcome criteria defining the expected general goal to be achieved

- Listing of interventions with rationales that include actions that may be performed for all of the related or risk factors identified for the diagnosis and applicable to any cross-referenced condition as well as the conditions included in the system

- Information, Instruction, Demonstration including interventions and rationales that pertain to the teaching function of the nurse

- Discharge or Maintenance Evaluation including specific behaviors expected of the client as a result of the interventions planned to achieve the desired outcomes

Each condition within the systems includes an Introductory paragraph that provides information about the condition in relation to the older adult, a Pathophysiological flow sheet depicting causative factors, pathology, resultant signs and symptoms and complications, Medical care that lists possible medications prescribed for the condition(s), and drug action, diagnostic procedures, laboratory tests and expected results, Nursing care plan that includes the Essential nursing diagnoses with specific related factors or risks and defining characteristics as they relate to this condition taken from the system essential diagnoses and plans (these are referenced so that the developed plan may be used in this condition), followed by the Specific nursing diagnoses, related or risk factors, defining characteristics and a developed plan using the same format as the essential diagnoses and care plans.

Since it is not uncommon for the elderly client to have more than one medical condition that requires treatment and care or that one condition may contribute to the existence or development of another medical problem, it may be necessary to combine the plans or use those portions of the plans that are applicable to an individual client. It is hoped that the practitioner will find these plans to be flexible enough to accomplish this interrelationship among the nursing diagnoses and care options.

Table of Contents

Cardiovascular System

Cardiovascular System

Cardiovascular disease is the leading pathophysiological condition in the geriatric client and is the leading cause of death in those over 65 years of age. The effectiveness of the pumping action of the heart and transporting function of the vascular system are influenced by organic changes that take place during the aging process. These changes create or contribute to alterations in the system that lead to disease, dysfunction or both. Cardiac parameters of the aging heart depend on changes in heart structure and function, physiological changes and electrocardiographic changes. Vascular parameters of the aging arteries, veins and capillaries depend on changes in collagen. elastin ratio, vasopressor control, venous muscle tone, valve function and capillary permeability. Under normal conditions, the aging heart adapts and allows for the average activities of the elderly. Anatomic and physiologic changes result in reduced stroke volume and cardiac output. This will cause difficulty in adaptation of the heart to the additional workload when demands of an illness (hypertension, myocardial infarction, valvular disease) are made on it.

GENERAL CARDIOVASCULAR CHANGES ASSOCIATED WITH THE AGING PROCESS

Heart, endocardium and valve structure

- Cardiac atrophy resulting from chronic illness and decreased activity (immobility) causing a decrease in heart size.
- Hemodynamic stress in aging causing a thickening and sclerosing of the endocardium.
- Hemodynamic stress in aging causing a thickening and rigidity of the valves especially the mitral and aortic valves which results in inaccurate closing and murmur sounds on auscultation and increased resistance to blood flow.
- Kyphosis/scoliosis may cause heart displacement.

Vascular structure

- Gradual increase in amount of connective tissue and decrease in elastin in connective tissue (collagen-elastin ratio) causing progressive stiffness and increase in the size of intramuscular veins and large muscular arteries; heart valves, endocardium and left ventricle become thicker.
- Aortic lengthening and sclerotic changes causing soft, systolic murmurs on auscultation.
- Increasing arterial thickening and loss of elasticity causing increased resistance to compression as in taking a pulse.
- Increasing changes in arterial walls (atherosclerosis) causing calcification and reduced lumen size; occlusion of coronary arteries leading to circulation abnormalities.
- Decreased effectiveness of venous valves and muscle tone causing reduced return of blood to the heart.
- Progressive inactivity causing distended superficial veins creating a high incidence of varicosities.
- Loss of subcutaneous fat causing increased response to cool environment with extremities cool to touch.

Physiological function of heart and transport function of vessels

- The work of the left ventricle and blood pumped by the heart at rest decreases causing a reduction in cardiac output of less than the normal 4-8L/minute.
- Decreased left ventricle compliance causing S_4 sounds on auscultation in some elderly.
- Cardiac reserve diminishes and is less capable in response to increasing demands causing poor reaction to stress.
- Decreased blood flow through coronary arteries of about 35% at 60 years of age.
- Loss of muscle fibers in the heart from increased collagen around fibers causing reduced contractility and filling capacity.
- Delayed recovery of contractility and irritability of myocardium causing poor response to tachycardia.
- Decreased ability of heart to utilize oxygen causing oxygen/activity imbalance and inadequate supply of oxygen to heart (ischemia).
- Decreased capillary permeability (capillary basement membranes thicken) affecting transport of nutrients and oxygen to tissues and removal of waste products from tissues.
- Loss of elasticity in walls of arteries (intima and media) and increased lability of vasopressor control causing decreased ability to stretch or expand and changes in blood pressure.
- Both systolic and diastolic increase slightly up to 70 years of age.
- Systolic increases faster than diastolic causing a widening of pulse pressure.
- Systolic increases with exercise and takes longer to return to baseline.
- An increase in peripheral resistance from arteriole constriction causing an increase in systolic and diastolic blood pressure increasing the workload of the heart.
- Infrequent ectopic beats in some elderly on auscultation; increase in variability of pulse rate.
- Increased vagal tone causing decrease in heart/ pulse rate.
- Reduced sensitivity to pressure changes by the baroreceptors in the aorta and carotid arteries causing slow response to postural changes.

Electrocardiograph changes

- Cellular changes, fibrosis of conduction system, neurogenic effect that impairs vasomotor response of vessels may cause minor changes in ECG; prolonged intervals may be evident from a slowdown of the conduction system (QRS, PR and QT); also left axis deviation and possibly decreased voltage of all waves.

ESSENTIAL NURSING DIAGNOSES AND CARE PLANS

Decreased cardiac output

Related to: Alteration in preload, alteration in afterload, alteration in inotropic (contractility) changes in heart
Defining characteristics: Variations in BP and pulse, fatigue, change in color, cold, clammy skin; decreased peripheral pulse, jugular vein distention, oliguria, dependent edema, dyspnea, orthopnea, crackles, hypoxia, restlessness

Related to: Alteration in rate, alteration in rhythm, alteration in conduction
Defining characteristics: Variations in external hemodynamics (VS), dysrrhythmias: ECG changes, gallop rhythm

Outcome Criteria

Return to and maintenance of stable BP, pulse rate, rhythm and respiratory parameters within baseline levels; prevention of irreversible complications associated with reduced cardiac output.

Interventions	Rationales
Assess level of cardiac functioning and existing cardiac and other conditions	Changes associated with aging are the cause of cardiac conditions; the existence of other factors additional burden on the heart
Assess BP, pulse rate and rhythm, apical pulse, respiratory rate, depth and ease (dyspnea), cough, hemoptysis, mentation changes, skin color and temperature	Indication of reduced cardiac output, vasodilation, lower blood volume if BP is increased (afterload), pulse rate increased (contractility and conduction). Pulse decreases may be associated with digitalis toxicity. Respiratory changes or difficulties that decrease oxygen in take and cause hypoxia (contractility); preload depends on venous return of blood to heart, afterload on resistance against which the heart must pump blood; contractility or ability of myocardium to adjust the force of contractions
Auscultate heart sounds for S_3 or S_4, gallop or murmur; breath sounds for crackles, wheezes	Reveals mechanical or electrical alterations in cardiac function
Assess existence of dysrrhythmias, change in PR interval per ECG tracings	The heart conduction system (specialized pacemaker cells) controls the rhythmic contractions and relaxations of the heart and maintains its pumping efficiency, rate and rhythm which ultimately affects cardiac output (afterload)

Interventions	Rationales
Assess lower extremities, sacral area for edema, distended neck veins, cold hands and feet, oliguria	Indication of reduced venous return to the heart and low cardiac output; oliguria is the result of decreased venous return caused by fluid retention resulting in reduced urinary output
Administer cardiac glycosides, nitrates, vasodilators, antihypertensives, diuretics and K replacement if needed	Treats vasoconstriction, reduces heart rate and contractility, reduces blood pressure, relaxes venous and arterial vessels which acts to in crease cardiac output and decrease work of heart
Position in semi-Fowler's or orthopneic	Prevents pooling of blood in pulmonary vessels and facilitates breathing
Weigh daily on same scale, same time	Weight gain indicates fluid retention
Pace activities avoiding going past point of tolerance and progress in exercise regimen as able	Prevents undue demands on heart and protects cardiac function by preventing sudden reduction in cardiac output
Avoid Valsalva maneuver with straining, coughing or moving	Results in sudden reduction in cardiac output by increasing intraabdominal and intrathoracic pressures preventing blood from entering thoracic cavity with less pumped into the heart, heart rate slows and cardiac output decreases; a sudden overload of blood to heart follows relaxation and decreased thoracic pressure

Information, Instruction, Demonstration

Interventions	Rationales
Administration of prescribed medications, actions and side effects; avoid over-the-counter drugs without physician advice	Promotes desired action and results; prevents adverse interactions with other drugs; drugs detoxify more slowly if hepatic congestion develops
Program of activities; active and passive ROM	Promotes circulation by preserving muscle tone and strength; heat generated by exercises promotes cellular permeability
Established pattern of bowel elimination of soft stool; proper administration of stool softener or laxative	Promotes easy elimination without straining
Elevate legs when sitting, avoid standing in one place or for long periods of time	Promotes venous blood return
Report edema, chest pain, changes in VS output, I&O imbalance	May indicate complications of reduced cardiac output
Technique for taking pulse and blood pressure	Allows for self-monitoring

Discharge or Maintenance Evaluation

- BP, pulse and respirations within baseline levels, breath sounds clear with optimal airflow, palpable peripheral pulses, absence of dyspnea
- Reduction of fatigue with increased activity tolerance
- Improved urinary output, absence of edema, absense of chest pain
- Skin warm, dry and color within normal tone
- Weight at baseline level

- Correct administration of medications with desired effect achieved

Altered tissue perfusion: cerebral, cardiopulmonary, gastrointestinal, renal, peripheral

Related to: Interruption of arterial flow
Defining characteristics: *Peripheral:* Skin cold, blue or purple color in dependent position, pale on elevation of extremity, diminished arterial pulses; slow growing, dry, thick, brittle nails; claudication, bruits, BP changes in extremities; slow healing of lesions. *Cerebral:* Changes in carotid pulses, carotid bruits, confusion, changes in mentation, cloudiness, restlessness, lethargy, stupor, depressed tendon reflex, tremors. *Cardiopulmonary:* BP and pulse changes, ABG changes in O_2 level and CO_2 level, cyanosis, chest pain, dyspnea, ventilation perfusion imbalance. *Renal:* Oliguria, anuria, dependent edema, electrolyte imbalance

Related to: Interruption of venous flow
Defining characteristics: Aching pain in extremities, pain in calf; heaviness with prolonged sitting, standing; skin discoloration, tissue congestion, edema, swelling; impaired tissue nutrition, oxygenation; positive Homan's sign; stasis dermatitis, ulcer

Outcome Criteria

Preservation of blood flow and perfusion to vital organs by optimal circulatory function.

Interventions	Rationales
Assess functional abilities in relation to affected system(s); nutrition, elimination, breathing pattern, mental function	Interrelationships of systems cause an overlapping of signs and symptoms associated with changes in tissue perfusion as related to specific organ function and transport system affected (arterial or venous)

Interventions	Rationales
Assess VS in three positions, arterial pulses, capillary refill time, changes in skin color, bilateral inequalities of temperature, dry and shiny skin, hair on legs, thick nails of feet, changes in mentation, urinary output, dyspnea, cyanosis, bruits, dependent edema	Signs and symptoms of reduced arterial tissue perfusion which are system dependent
Assess extremities for feeling of heaviness and aching from prolonged standing, skin discoloration, dermatitis, edema or swelling and deep muscle tenderness in leg calf, visible enlarged veins	Signs and symptoms of reduced venous circulation associated with increased venous pressure, incompetent valves and impaired emptying; inflammation of veins, thrombus formation
Administer vasodilator, anticoagulant, antiplatelet agent, antilipidemic, cardiac gycoside, analgesic	Treats vasoconstriction, inhibits blood clotting, decreases RBC and platelet aggregation, prevents synthesis of cholesterol and reduces blood level, controls pain all of which enhances blood flow
Encourage ambulation and exercises, active or passive ROM	Promotes peripheral arterial circulation and prevents venous stasis
Elevate legs at heart level or below heart	Promotes arterial flow
Provide protectors to bony prominences, foot cradle	Prevents pressure to extremities with poor circulation and tissue perfusion
Apply elastic hose; elevate legs when sitting	Promotes venous return
Provide O_2 by cannula with rate based on ABGs and disease/condition	Provides oxygen necessary to tissues and organs for proper functioning

Interventions	Rationales
Maintain reality orientation and protect preservation of mental disoriented	Provides caring, support, protection and from injury if confused or capacities

Information, Instruction, Demonstration

Interventions	Rationales
Avoid exposure to cold environment; wear warm clothing	Causes vasoconstriction, decreased circulation and perfusion
Avoid hot baths, hot application to feet, scratching feet	May cause burns if tactile perception is impaired as circulation is reduced
Wear protective shoes and clean well-fitting socks	Protects feet from injury
Avoid wearing tight clothing or jewelry, garters, crossing legs	Constricts circulation and reduces venous return
Administration of prescribed medications, actions and side effects	Promotes correct administration of drugs and desired effects
Refrain from smoking	Causes vasoconstriction
Menu planning to reduce fat, cholesterol, salt content	Reduces cholesterol levels to control atherosclerosis and effect on blood flow
Schedule and plan for rest and activity based on pain and fatigue	Prevents fatigue while promoting circulation and increased work of heart

Discharge or Maintenance Evaluation

- Lungs clear with absence of adventitious sounds
- Extremities warm, normal color with equal palpable pulses
- VS returned to baseline levels for age/sex

- Performs regular exercises
- Absence of ulcerations on legs, tissue injury as result of trauma prevented
- Reduced pressure on skin, avoids prolonged standing, crossing legs
- Statements that pain reduced or controlled with medication or rest
- Resolution of cerebral hypoxemia with return of baseline mental capacity and behaviors
- Urinary output in balance with intake, absence of edema, thirst, dry skin, poor turgor
- Compliance with low fat, cholesterol and salt diet with lipid panel revealing reduced levels of cholesterol, triglycerides, LDL

Fluid volume excess

Related to: Compromised regulatory mechanisms
Defining characteristics: Edema, weight gain, effusion, shortness of breath, orthopnea, crackles on auscultation, change in respiratory pattern, blood pressure changes, jugular vein distention, oliguria, specific gravity changes, altered electrolytes, azoturia

Related to: Excessive sodium intake
Defining characteristics: Weight gain, edema, intake greater than output, blood pressure changes (increased)

Outcome Criteria

Minimal or absence of fluid retention or edema in all body parts and BP, I&O within baseline ranges maintained.

Interventions	Rationales
Assess presence of dependent edema (pedal and sacral), daily weight gain, increases in circumference of the extremities or abdomen, jugular vein distension	Edema is the excess accumulation of interstitial fluid in the tissues or organs caused by increased capillary pressure or permeability associated with decreased resistance to flow through arterioles, increased resistance to flow through venules or loss of capillary wall integrity or by decreased osmotic pressure to move fluid from the tissue back into the capillaries; weight gain of 1 lb/day indicates fluid retention (5 lb = 2 L fluid)
Assess lungs for crackles, diminished breath sounds, dyspnea, orthopnea, dry, non-productive cough, hemoptysis, heart sounds for crackles, pulse rate	Indicates pulmonary fluid retention (effusion, pulmonary edema) and failure of renal regulation is associated with rduced cardiac output
Assess for hepatomegaly, anasarca, splenomegaly	Generalized body edema that may be associated with some heart or renal conditions
Assess for oliguria, increased specific gravity, electrolyte imbalances, intake greater than output	Indicates decreased renal perfusion with sodium and potassium retention
Administer diuretic therapy and maintain I&O flow sheet to ensure an output of at least 30 ml/hr; monitor for hypokalemia resulting from diuresis	Monitors I&O ratio to ensure renal function and potassium loss and need for replacement during therapy to remove fluid excess; excessive potassium losses may lead to ECG changes

Interventions	Rationales
Restrict movement/ activity, elevate legs, pad areas and bony prominences, change position q2h	Edematous tissue interferes with movement and is more susceptible to injury from pressure; edematous tissue is not well oxygenated and suffers from reduced circulation of nutrients and removal of wastes; limited activity and bed-rest reduces oxygen needs
Monitor I&O to include urine, emesis, feces, diaphoresis in output and all fluid intake via all routes	Evaluate fluid balance to determine excesses and losses
Restrict fluids and dietary sodium, reduce calories if overweight	High salt intake can cause fluid retention

Information, Instruction, Demonstration

Interventions	Rationales
Menu planning for low sodium diet (2 Gm sodium diet). Offer lists of food selections, information about seasonings and commercially prepared foods to avoid	Reduces fluid and electrolyte retention
Daily weight on same scale, at same time wearing same clothing; report gains and losses	Provides information about weight gain indicating fluid retention
Administration of diuretic and fluid intake if restricted, dietary intake of foods containing K	Treats edema by excretion of fluid and replaces K losses
Wear proper fitting shoes and clothing	Edema may create tightness

Interventions	Rationales
Avoid prolonged standing, hot environment, sudden change in position from sitting or lying to standing	Predisposes to increased capillary pressure by effects of gravity and increased vascular volume (dilatation of superficial vessels); prevents falls due to orthostatic hypotension
Pacing of activities with gradual increases when appropriate	Promotes circulation

Discharge or Maintenance Evaluation

- VS returned to baseline levels/ranges
- Peripheral and organ edema reduced or eliminated with abdominal and extremity circumference returned to baseline measurements
- Weight maintained with less than 1 lb deviation
- I&O ratio maintained
- Proper administration of diuretic; statements of action, side effects, amount and frequency
- Compliance with reduced sodium diet; 24 hr menu planned with fluid distribution

Coronary Artery Disease

Genetic factors

Diabetes mellitus

Hypertension

Increased lipids, cholesterol, triglycerides

Environmental factors: obesity, smoking, stress, lack of activity

↓ ↓ ↓ ↓ ↓

Coronary atherosclerosis

↓

Coronary artery disease

↓

75% obstruction of blood flow through coronary arteries, inadequate collateral circulation

↓ ↓

Myocardial thrombosis

Myocardial ischemia

↓ ↓

Death of myocardial tissue

Metabolic needs more than than blood flow delivers

↓ ↓

Acute myocardial infarction

Substernal or precordial pain radiating to shoulder, jaw or down left arm
Dyspnea
Substernal pressure

↓ ↓

May have precordial pain
Dyspnea
Decreased BP, tachycardia, palpitations
Nausea, vomiting, hiccups
Weakness, fatigue in arms and legs
Fever, leukocytosis

Persistent unstable angina

↓ ↓

Dysrhythmias
Congestive heart failure

Myocardial infarction

Coronary Artery Disease

A condition associated with the aging process because of its relationship with coronary atherosclerosis. A major cause of heart disease in the elderly population, abnormal consequences of the condition depend on development of collateral circulation to compensate for the degree of coronary atherosclerosis. If the atherosclerosis and narrowing of the arteries is greater than the ability of collateral circulation to bypass points of obstruction, signs and symptoms of CAD appear. These depend on the extent of CAD and cerebral damage. The major abnormality resulting from CAD is angina pectoris which may lead to myocardial infarction if persistent or unstable.

MEDICAL CARE

Analgesics: morphine (MS) IM to decrease neuro-transmitter release used for myocardial infarction pain

Antianginal nitrates/nitrites: nitroglycerin SL, ointment (Nitrol), transdermal (Nitro-Dur); PO, sustained release isosorbide dinitrate (Isordil) to relieve angina pain by dilating coronary arteries and peripheral blood vessels

Antianginal, beta-adrenergic blocker: propranolol (Inderal) PO to decrease myocardial contractility, heart rate and peripheral resistance; decrease oxygen demands of heart

Antianginal, calcium channel blocker: nifedipine (Procardia) PO to decrease systemic vascular resistance, cardiac contractility and promote coronary vasodilatation

Stool softners: docusate sodium (Colace) PO to lower surface tension and allow water to soften stool in colon for elimination without straining

Antianxieties: alprazolam (Xanax) PO for anxiety reduction by action at limbic and subcortical levels of CNS

Anticoagulants: warfarin (Coumadin) PO for myocardial infarction to prevent extension of thrombi and development of additional clots

Antiplatelet agent: aspirin PO to prevent platelet aggregation

Antilipidemics: cholestyramine (Questran) PO lowers cholesterol in gastrointestinal tract and inhibits its absorption, clofibrate (Atromide-S) PO lowers triglyceride levels by inhibiting synthesis of lipids, niacin (Slo-Niacin) PO decreases blood lipids

Chest x-ray: Reveals cardiac enlargement, calcifications, pulmonary congestion if present

Exercise stress test (with or without radionuclides): Reveals disease process (coronary artery obstruction) if age allows for exercise

Electrocardiography (12 lead): Reveals changes indicating past myocardial infarction or changes when compared to past ECG

Positron emission tomography: Reveals ischemia and infarction

Nuclear imaging: Using radionuclide reveals myocardial perfusion

Cardiac catheterization: Reveals presence of CAD to evaluate pressures, oxygen level, and cardiac output

Lipid panel: Reveals levels of lipoproteins (HDL, LDL), cholesterol, triglycerides

Enzymes (CDK, AST, LDH): Increased levels indicate cardiac damage, increased CK-MB and LDH-1 isoenzymes

CBC: Increased levels in WBC if myocardial infarction occured

Electrolytes: Na, Cl, K for increased or decreased levels

NURSING CARE PLANS

Essential nursing diagnoses and plans associated with this condition:

Decreased cardiac output (4)

Related to: Alteration in preload, afterload, inotropic changes in heart from increased systemic vascular resistance and decreased myocardial contractility

Defining characteristics: BP and pulse changes (initially elevated and then BP drops as cardiac output decreases and pulse increases), change in color and cold, clammy skin, oliguria, jugular vein distention, dyspnea, crackles, edema (peripheral or dependent)

Related to: Alteration in rate, rhythm, conduction from decreased coronary blood flow (ischemia) to myocardial tissue

Defining characteristics: Variations in BP and pulse, arrhythmias, ECG changes in T and Q waves, ST segment, distant heart sounds, abnormal S_3 and S_4 (gallop rhythm)

Altered tissue perfusion: cardiopulmonary (6)

Related to: Interruption of arterial flow to myocardial tissue reducing oxygen supply from infarction, spasms, stenosis of coronary artery

Defining characteristics: Chest pain, dyspnea, crackles, ventilation perfusion imbalance

Impaired gas exchange (47)

Related to: Ventilation perfusion imbalance from ineffective breathing pattern and fluid in lungs, ineffective ventricular function

Defining characteristics: Exertional dyspnea, tachypnea, hypoxia, crackles, hypercapna, activities intolerance

SPECIFIC DIAGNOSES AND CARE PLANS

Pain

Related to: Biological injuring agents (myocardial ischemia)

Defining characteristics: Communication of verbal pain descriptors; chest pain radiating to arm, jaw or neck; clutching at chest in MI; chest pain precipitated by activity, intermittent and radiating to left arm in angina; diaphoresis; clenching fists; dyspnea; dizziness

Outcome Criteria

Pain relief in 5-10 seconds with reduced angina episodes. Pain relieved and controlled in presence of MI.

Interventions	Rationales
Assess characteristics of pain, precipitating factors, verbal and nonverbal responses, pain onset, location, severity, duration, and radiating	Pain from angina occurs when myocardial need for oxygen exceeds ability of coronary vessels to supply needed blood flow as lumen is narrowed by athero sclerosis and, in MI blood flow is obstructed by thrombosis in coronary artery causing death of myocardial tissue
Monitor VS during pain episode	Increases in pulse and BP caused by anxiety, stress precipitates angina episode
Administer analgesic, morphine (MS) IM or vasodilator, nitroglycerin SL; repeat nitroglycerin if pain not relieved in 5 min	Morphine given to control MI pain and nitroglycerin to control angina pain
Administer O_2 at 2-4 L/min. via nasal cannula	Relieves heart muscle hypoxia

Interventions	Rationales
Maintain rest during angina attack; stay with client	Reduces oxygen need and promotes caring attitude and trust
Limit activity and maintain bedrest in presence of MI	Decreases myocardial oxygen consumption and strain on heart
Maintain quiet, calm environment, provide relaxing backrub, guided imagery	Reduces stimuli that increases oxygen demand

Information, Instruction, Demonstration

Interventions	Rationales
Report pain lasting longer than 15 min.; review effect of medication administration	Indication that medication adjustment needs to be made or cardiac complication present
Maintain log of time, duration and location of angina episodes, amount of medication taken	Offers comparisons for physician to review
Avoid activities that precipitate angina episodes such as sudden exposure to cold, drinking cold liquids, stressful situations, large meals, straining at stools, cigarette smoking, caffeine containing beverages	Reduces frequency of attacks

Discharge or Maintenance Evaluation

- Statements that pain is absent or relieved with medication administration
- Administers medication before pain becomes severe, repeats medication as prescribed

- Behavior that precipitates angina episode is modified

Anxiety

Related to: Threat of death (life-threatening crisis of heart attack or impending heart attack)
Defining characteristics: Communication of apprehension, sense of impending doom, fear of unspecific consequences, restlessness, anxious, worried

Related to: Threat to change in health status (angina attacks, limitations in activity)
Defining characteristics: Communication of uncertainty, concerns regarding changes in life events, feelings of inadequacy, helplessness

Outcome Criteria

Anxiety level reduced and maintained at acceptable level.

Interventions	Rationales
Assess changes in anxiety level during periods of pain or changes in respirations, verbalizations of fear, sense of doom	Anxiety results in increased oxygen demand on an already impaired heart
Provide calm, supportive environment for expression of fears, concerns change in health status	Reduces anxiety and promotes rapport, caring and trust and feelings about
Encourage visits from family, friends	Provides emotional support
Speak in low voice, slowly and quietly	Prevents additional stimuli
Administer sedative, antianxiety agent with caution	Promotes relaxation and reduces anxiety; elderly very sensitive to effects of sedation as drug metabolism is slower and effects more profound

Information, Instruction, Demonstration

Interventions	Rationales
Inform that angina is not a heart attack and that the pain from ischemia is reversible	Allays anxiety and fear
New methods in treating MI successful in preventing complications and dissolving clot	Reduces fear of death

Discharge or Maintenance Evaluation

- Statements that anxiety is reduced
- Performs relaxation exercises when exposed to stress
- Avoids stressful visitors, telephone calls or other provoking events

Activity intolerance

Related to: Imbalance between oxygen supply and demand (myocardial ischemia)
Defining characteristics: Chest pain, dyspnea, increased pulse and BP during activity

Outcome Criteria

Optimal activity level with increased energy and endurance within imposed restrictions.

Interventions	Rationales
Assess baseline tolerance for activity, ability to adapt to limitations and/ or restrictions on lifestyle	Promotes, protects circulatory function and reduces cardiac workload

Interventions	Rationales
Assess pulse, respiration, BP 5 min before, during and after activity	Pulse increase more than 20/min and increases in BP and respirations indicates need for reduction in activity
If activity causes pain, administer vasodilator (nitroglycerin) SL 5 min before	Controls pain during activity whether part of rehabilitation or sexual activity
Provide progressive activity following bedrest to allow to use commode, sit at side of bed, sit in chair, ambulate as client is able	Allows for activity program that increases slowly as endurance increases
Schedule activities around rest periods	Maintains activity below angina threshold

Information, Instruction, Demonstration

Interventions	Rationales
Avoid extending activities beyond tolerance	Conserves energy and prevents angina episode
Avoid activity after eating, bathing or during stress periods	Requires additional oxygen
Keep medication nearby when performing activity	Availability to administer when needed
Inform to cease activity when pain occurs and when taking medication, sit on chair and wait for pain to pass	Prevents falls if feeling dizzy or faint; decreases O_2 requirement
Suggest cardiac rehabilitation program to establish a daily acceptable exercise plan within determined limits	Provides necessary activity without causing increased workload to heart and pain episode; improves circulation

Interventions	Rationales
Inform to rest by sitting in chair rather than lying in bed, conserve energy during activities	Preferred position for rest; prevents complications associated with immobility and prevents pooling of blood in pulmonary vessels

Discharge or Maintenance Evaluation

- Absence of pain during activity
- Participates in ADL, sexual activity within established restrictions
- Participates in daily exercise program as during optional therapy level allows for adequate rest
- Statements that feeling less weak and energy level increased
- Administers medication properly and reports persistent pain after initial and two additional doses of nitroglycerin
- Statements that identify difference between activity intolerance caused by angina attack and MI onset

Altered sexuality pattern

Related to: Knowledge deficit about alternative responses to health-related transitions, altered body function (angina episode or fear of recurring MI during activity)
Defining characteristics: Verbalization of difficulties, limitations, or changes in sexual behaviors or activities

Outcome Criteria

Satisfying adjustments made in sexual activity that result in positive sexual experience.

Interventions	Rationales
Assess desire and comfort in discussing concerns about sexual activity	May be embarrassed or not know how to approach the subject
Discuss feelings of inadequacy or fear of sexual function; correct misinformation	May fear precipitating angina episode or heart attack
Use exercise tolerance, changes in VS caused by activity as guideline to develop a plan of progressive sexual activity based on physical limits	Provides activity without symptoms that create fear or interfere with sexual activity
Include partner in discussion and plan	May desire to discuss alone or with partner present

Information, Instruction, Demonstration

Interventions	Rationales
Inform about the effects of medications that affect libido and sexual function	Medications often affect sexual function and cause unsatisfactory experience
Instruct to take the medications before sexual activity	Prevents anginal episode
Instruct that increased pulse and respiration for 15 min or longer after intercourse should be reported	Provides for adjustments in medication, positioning or other factors to prevent complication
Refer to sex therapist for assistance as appropriate	Provides alternatives for satisfying experience

Discharge or Maintenance Evaluation

- Pulse, respiration increases within determined ranges after intercourse
- Administers medications before sexual activity
- Verbalizes satisfying sexual experience within limitations
- Consults sex therapist or counselor if needed

Knowledge deficit

Related to: Lack of information and cognitive skills (CAD and risk of cardiovascular disease, medical regimen for angina and MI)
Defining characteristics: Verbalization of the problem, inaccurate follow-through of instructions, request for information, apathetic behavior

Outcome Criteria

Knowledge of medical regimen, risk factors for angina, MI, CAD; compliance with preventive regimen.

Interventions	Rationales
Assess knowledge of causes/risk factors associated with disease and methods to control angina, medical regimen for MI	Prevents repetition of information; promotes compliance with medical regimen to prevent extension of CAD and consequences of heart disease
Provide explanations and information in clear, simple language that is understandable; provide limited amounts of information over periods of time rather than large amounts at one sitting	Enhances compliance related to cognitive abilities, sensory deficits
Use pamphlets, videotapes, teaching aids with consideration for neurosensory deficits	Reinforces learning and increases understanding and compliance

Interventions	Rationales
Assist to plan low sodium, fat, cholesterol; reduction diet if overweight or refer to nutritionist for assistance	Provides for reduction in risk factors contributing to heart disease
Assist with exercise program following cardiac rehabilitation for daily isotonic activities	Provides for optimal circulation without danger of cardiac damage or dysfunction
Inform about medication administration including dose, when to take, frequency, method of taking, side effects and what to report, expected results; use color-coded or labeled pill container, pill crusher, other aids as needed	Ensures accurate medication dosages and desired effect
Avoid over-the-counter drugs without physician consent, cigarette smoking	May interact with prescribed drugs

Discharge or Maintenance Evaluation

- Statements of knowledge and correct administration of medications
- Weight within baseline parameters; loss of 1 lb/week if desired
- Perform daily isotonic exercises; schedule dependent on abilities
- Limits smoking, alcohol intake
- Plans and/or ingests 3-6 meals/day of low sodium, fat and cholesterol content; statements of what foods to include and avoid
- Statements of causes and risk factors associated with CAD, MI

Heart Failure

A common complication of heart conditions that increases with aging, heart failure is the inability of the heart to pump adequate amounts of blood to fulfill the metabolic needs of body tissues. It may be right-sided or left-sided with both sides involved in heart failure that is present over long periods of time. Age determines the severity of manifestations found in chronic heart failure along with the type and severity of heart disease present.

MEDICAL CARE

Cardiac glycosides: digitalis (Digoxin) PO to increase force and strength of ventricular contractions (inotropic) and to decrease conduction and rate of contractions (chronotropic) which increases cardiac output

Diuretics: furosemide (Lasix), hydrochlorothiazide (Exidrex) PO to promote fluid removal and excretion to reduce edema and pulmonary venous pressure by preventing sodium and water reabsorption

Vasodilators: hydralazine (Apresoline) PO to relax arterial smooth muscle; isosorbide dinitrate (Isordil) SL or PO to relax venous smooth muscle; prazosin (Minipress) to relax both arterial and venous smooth muscle

Renin-angiotensin antagonists: captopril (Capoten) PO to prevent the conversion of angiotensin I to II to reduce vasoconstriction and work of the heart (reduce preload and afterload)

Electrolytes: potassium bicarbonate (K-Lyte) PO to replace potassium lost in diuretic therapy

Chest x-ray: Reveals enlargement of heart and pulmonary vein; pleural effusion in pulmonary edema

Electrocardiography: Reveals changes associated with ventricular enlargement, arrhythmias

Echocardiography: Reveals chamber size and ventricular activity

Electrolytes: K, Na, Cl, Ca, Mg, P, HCO_3 for imbalances affecting heart function

Enzymes: CPK, CK-MB, LDH revealing cardiac damage

Anticoagulant levels: PT, PTT revealing desired response to therapy

CBC: RBC, MCH, MCHC, Hb revealing hematologic abnormalities

Albumin, total proteins: revealing nutritional status

ABGs: revealing hypoxemia, hypercapnia

NURSING CARE PLANS

Essential nursing diagnoses and plans associated with this condition:

Decreased cardiac output (4)

Related to: Alteration in preload, afterload, inotropic changes in heart from accumulation of blood in lungs or systemic venous system
Defining characteristics: Variations in BP and pulse, fatigue, cold, clammy skin, cyanosis, dependent edema, dyspnea, orthopnea, cough, crackles, ascites, hepatomegaly, splenomegaly, frothy, bloody sputum, confusion, nocturia, restlessness

Heart Failure

Right Sided Heart Failure	**Left Sided Heart Failure**

Right Sided Heart Failure

Pulmonary hypertension
COPD (cor pulmonale)
Anemia
Thyrotoxicosis

↓

Accumulation of bood in systemic venous system

↓

Increased right arterial and peripheral venous pressure

↓

Right-sided failure

↓

Peripheral edema (sacral and lower extremeties)
Congestion of portal circulation (lever, spleen)

↓

Weight gain
Anorexia
Acites, abdominal pain
Fatigue
Cyanosis

Left Sided Heart Failure

Hypertension
Mycardial infarction
Valvular heart disease
Arrhythmias
Anemia

↓

Accumulation of blood in lungs

↓

Congestion of pulmonary circulation

↓

Increased pulmonary capillary pressure

↓

Left-sided failure

↓

Pulmonary edema (fluid moves into alveoli)

↓

Congestive heart failure

↓

Impaired gas exchange

↓

Cyanosis
Dyspenea, orthopnea
Cough, nocturia

Advanced heart failure   ←   ↓

↓

Air hunger/gasping
Tachycardia/cackles
Frothy, blood-tinged
sputum
Skin moist, cool
Cyanosis lips, nail beds
Confusion stupor   ←   Advanced heart
failure in aged

↓

Insomnia
Anxiety
Restlessness
Confusion

Fluid volume excess (8)

Related to: Compromised regulatory mechanisms of heart's failure to act as a pump and maintain cardiac output
Defining characteristics: Edema, weight gain, effusion, dyspnea, orthopnea, crackles, oliguria, change in respiratory pattern, ascites, peripheral edema, hepatomegaly, splenomegaly, cyanosis, frothy, blood-tinged sputum, confusion, restlessness

Impaired gas exchange (47)

Related to: Ventilation perfusion imbalance from fluid in alevoli and reduced area for exchange in left sided failure
Defining characteristics: Hypoxia, restlessness, somnolence, confusion, altered mentation, hypercapnea, cyanosis, dyspnea, crackles, activity intolerance

Constipation (121)

Related to: Less than adequate fluids, dietary intake and bulk, anorexia, gastrointestinal distress
Defining characteristics: Decreased appetite, abdominal pain, hepatomegaly, nausea, hard-formed stool, reduced frequency

Related to: Less than adequate physical activity or immobility from bedrest, fatigue
Defining characteristics: Activity intolerance, weakness, dyspnea

Sleep pattern disturbance (77)

Related to: Internal factors of illness from heart failure
Defining characteristics: Interrupted sleep, restlessness, irritability, verbal complaints of not feeling rested, paroxysmal nocturnal dyspnea

Risk for impaired skin integrity (246)

Related to: Internal factors of altered circulation
Defining characteristics: Edema, irritation of skin areas, reddened areas, imposed immobility (bedrest)

SPECIFIC DIAGNOSES AND CARE PLANS

Fatigue

Related to: States of discomfort (activity intolerance)
Defining characteristics: Dyspnea, work of breathing, statements of fatigue/ lack of energy, increase in physical complaints

Related to: Decreased metabolic energy production (decreased cardiac output)
Defining characteristics: Inability to maintain usual routines, decreased performance, perceived need for additional energy to accomplish routine tasks

Outcome Criteria

Performance of activities at optimal level with increased energy; fatigue controlled within limits set for independent ADL activity.

Interventions	Rationales
Assess baseline tolerance for activity, expression of fatigue, weakness, respiratory changes	Impaired circulation results in poor oxygenation of tissues and low cardiac output results in inability of body to absorb nutrients both of which contribute to low energy reserve and fatigue

Interventions	Rationales
Assess response to existing or new activity; assist to identify tolerable level of activity without fatigue	Provides baselines without causing symptoms of heart failure and promotes participation in planning
Maintain bedrest during symptomatic periods; progressively increase activity tolerance by independent movement in bed, active ROM, sitting up in bed, in chair, ambulating to bathroom with daily increases in distance	Decreases oxygen needs while promoting increasing activity without excessive energy expenditure
Assist with ADL activities based on expression of fatigue; allow to progress gradually, daily and incorporate ROM	Conserves energy while promoting independence and endurance in ADL
Plan for rest periods during day without interruptions	Rest needed to prevent depletion of energy; nocturia resulting from lying position at night which allows fluid to move from interstitial spaces to circulation causing diuresis, paroxysmal nocturnal dyspnea resulting from fluid reabsorption from dependent areas interferes with sleep
Terminate activity that increases respirations of more than 20/min, pulse of more than 120/min, causes palpitations, dyspnea, diaphoresis, extreme weakness and fatigue	Indication of activity intolerance and could exacerbate heart failure

Information, Instruction, Demonstration

Interventions	Rationales
Plan time to perform activity by resting after each step, i.e., wash face, rest, brush teeth, rest	Conserves energy and prevents fatigue
Avoid Valsava's maneuver, advise to exhale when moving	Increases intrathoracic pressure changing cardiac output parameters
Explore possible cardiac rehabilitation program for use of treadmill, stationary bicycle, wall hanging weights, barbell exercises	Regulated program of isotonic and isometric exercises improves circulatory and respiratory function resulting in increased energy and endurance

Discharge or Maintenance Evaluation

- Daily increases in self-care of ADL until completely independent
- Statements that fatigue decreased, energy and tolerance for activities increased
- Walks at prescribed pace for 30 minutes 3 times/week, lifts barbells 10 times each arm daily
- Schedules rest periods during day for 30 minutes-1 hour 2-3 times/day
- Sleep pattern returned to baseline as awakenings reduced

Ineffective individual coping

Related to: Multiple life changes (loss of independence, limitations on lifestyle, chronic disease)
Defining characteristics: Inability to meet basic needs, dependency, chronic fatigue, worry, anxiety, poor self-esteem, verbalization of inability to cope

Outcome Criteria

Anxiety, worry, fatigue reduced; increased independence in activities and decision making process.

Interventions	Rationales
Assess coping methods, use of defense mechanisms, feelings about lifestyle changes, any losses associated with illness, ability to ask for help	Allows for interventions that promote control over life and ability to cope with long term illness
Assist to identify positive defense mechanisms and promote their use; new behaviors to be learned	Use of defense mechanisms that have worked in past increases ability to cope and promotes self-esteem
Provide environment that allows for free expression of concerns and fears	Encourages trust and relieves anxiety and worry
Assist to set short and long term goals; provide positive feedback regarding progress and focus on abilities rather than disabilities	Promotes self-worth and responsibility

Information, Instruction, Demonstration

Interventions	Rationales
Inform that compliance with treatment regimen reduces risk factors	Maintains health status by preventing recurrence of acute episode
Refer to support group or counseling if appropriate; involve family members if client desires	Provides information and support from others with similar experiences
Teach relaxation techniques	Reduces stress and anxiety

Interventions	Rationales
Teach problem solving approaches and new ways or methods to adapt to chronic illness	Promotes coping ability with life style changes

Discharge or Maintenance Evaluation

- Uses appropriate coping mechanisms and problem solving methods in adapting to functional losses
- Asks for assistance when needed
- Seeks level of independence appropriate with activity tolerance and coping ability
- Statements that anxiety, worry are decreasing and feels more in control and capable of making decisions regarding health status and functional limitations

Knowledge deficit

Related to: Lack of information (dietary, activity and drug therapy)
Defining characteristics: Verbalization of the problem, request for information, noncompliance with medical regimen

Outcome Criteria

Compliance with low sodium diet, drug therapy, exercise regimen.

Interventions	Rationales
Assess knowledge of proper diet for low sodium intake, administration of cardiac glycosides, diuretics, other drugs ordered	Provides basis for teaching and avoids repetition of information

Interventions	Rationales
Utilize booklets, pictures, tapes, charts in teaching client and family	Aids in teaching by use video of visual adjuncts
Provide clear explanations and instruction in medication names, action, dosage, frequency, storage, how to take and expected results	Enhances compliance as complexity and number of medications increase
Report side effects of anorexia, nausea, vomiting, diarrhea, headache, fatigue, blurred vision, irregular and slow pulse	Signs and symptoms of digitalis toxicity
Take pulse before taking cardiac glycoside, omit dose and report if pulse below 60/min (50/min if taking beta blocking drug)	Bradycardia leads to arrhythmia or other cardiac complication
Avoid use of table salt, commercially prepared or convenience foods, cheese, snack foods, soy sauce, pickled foods, sodas, antacids that contain salt	Reduces salt intake and fluid retention as increased sodium levels decrease movement of fluid from cell to capillary circulation
Include citrus juices, bananas, broths, whole grains	Foods that contain potassium for replacement if diuretic therapy given
Season foods with lemon and spices	Replaces salt as seasoning

Interventions	Rationales
Report weakness, palpitations, fatigue, leg cramps, excessive thirst, 2 lb/day weight loss	Signs and symptoms of hypokalemia if on diuretic therapy
Refer to dietician if weight loss plan needed	Overweight increases work load of heart
Modify activities to meet rest needs	Prevents fatigue and increased oxygen need

Discharge or Maintenance Evaluation

- Daily exercises within determined limitations
- Absence of drug toxicity, hypokalemia signs and symptoms
- Appropriate administration of medications daily
- Pulse, respirations within baseline ranges
- Report signs and symptoms indicating change in cardiac status (pain dyspnea, edema, fatigue)
- Dietary compliance of reducing sodium intake to
- 3000-7000mg/day
- Statements of foods to include and foods to avoid
- Weight loss of 1 lb/wk if on reducing diet
- Verbalizes causes, risk factors of heart failure

Hypertension

Defined in the elderly population as isolated hypertension with a systolic pressure greater than 160 mm Hg (elevated) and a diastolic pressure lower than 90 mm Hg (normal) or primary (essential) hypertension occurring as normal predictable increases with maturity and growth resulting in a systolic pressure greater than 160 mm Hg (elevated) and a diastolic pressure greater than 90 mm Hg (elevated). It is considered one of the most prevalent and urgent problems of the elderly individual because of its effect on circulation in the brain, heart and kidneys and workload of the heart. Complications from hypertension accounts for over 50% of deaths in the U.S.

MEDICAL CARE

Diuretics: hydrochlorothiazide (Esidrex), spironolactone (Aldactone) PO to promote diuresis and elimination of sodium by preventing reabsorption

Vasodilators: hydralazine (Apresoline), minoxidil (Loniten) PO to relax smooth muscle of arterioles resulting in reduced peripheral resistance

Antihypertensives (beta-adrenergic blocker): propranolol (Inderal), metoprolol (Lopressor), nadolol (Corgard) PO to decrease blood pressure by inhibiting impulse through sympathetic pathways, decrease cardiac output, sympathetic stimulation and renin secretion by kidneys

Antihypertensives (calcium channel blocker): verapamil (Isoptin), nifedipine (Procardia) PO to reduce blood pressure

Antihypertensives (central-acting adrenergics): clonidine (Catopres), methyldopa (Aldomet) PO to decrease peripheral resistance to lower blood pressure

Antihypertensives (angiotensin-converting enzyme inhibitor): captopril (Capoten) PO to lower total peripheral resistance by inhibiting angiotensin-converting enzyme

Electrolytes: potassium bicarbonate (K-Lyte) PO to replace potassium lost in diuretic therapy

Chest x-ray: Reveals heart and aortic dilatation

Electrocardiography: Reveals cardiac status as baseline information

Lipid panel: Reveals lipoproteins, cholesterol and triglyceride levels and relationship to risk factor of atherosclerosis

Electrolytes: Reveals hypokalemia, hypernatremia during diuretic therapy

NURSING CARE PLANS

Essential nursing diagnoses and plans associated with this condition

Fluid volume excess (8)

Related to: Excessive sodium intake included in diet
Defining characteristics: Weight gain, blood pressure increases, intake greater than output

Related to: Compromised regulatory mechanisms in hemodynamic, neurologic, renal systems
Defining characteristics: Dull headache, vertigo, memory impairment, dyspnea, nocturia, increased BP, fluid retention

Risk for fluid volume deficit (151)

Related to: Active loss caused by medication (diuretic)
Defining characteristics: Increased urinary output greater than intake, weight loss (sudden), hypokalemia, dry skin, mucous membranes, decreased skin turgor, thirst

Hypertension

Aging process　　　　　　　　　　Genetic factors:　　　　　　　Environmental factors:
↓　　　　　　　　　　　　　　　　　Na, K intake　　　　　　　　alcohol intake,
　　　　　　　　　　　　　　　　　　　　　　　　　　　　　obesity, stress

Loss of elastic fibers in media
Increased collagen and calcium in
media
Artheroscloerosis in intima
↓　　　　　　　　　　　　　　　　　　　↓　　　　　　　　　　　　　　　　↓

Stiffness of aortic and
peripheral arteries
↓

Constriction of arterioles　　→　　　　　　　↓　　　　　←　　　　　↓
↓

Hemodynamic mechanisms　　　　　Neurologic mechanisms　　　　Renal mechanisms
↓　　　　　　　　　　　　　　　　　↓　　　　　　　　　　　　　↓
　　　　　　　　　　　　　　　　　　　　　　　　　　　　Blood-borne substances
　　　　　　　　　　　　　　　　　　　　　　　　　　　　　　↓

Increased total peripheral　　　　Decreased baroreceptor　　　Sympathetic stimulation
resistance　　　　　　　　　　sensitivity (sympathetic　　Angiotensin and aldeosterone
Increased cardiac output　　　　nervous system deficit)　　　　release
↓　　　　　　　　　　　　　　　　　↓　　　　　　Decreased renal blood flow
　　　　　　　　　　　　　　　　　　　　　　　　　　　　　　↓

Impaired nutrition and　　　　　Changes in CSF pressure　　　Ischemia of renal tissue
oxygenation of myocardium
Increased workload of heart
↓　　　　　　　　　　　　　　　　　↓　　　　　　　　　　　　　↓

Dyspnea on exertion　　　　　　Memory impairment　　　　　　Nocturia
↓　　　　　　　　　　　　　Dull headache in AM　　　　Water and Na retention
　　　　　　　　　　　　　　　　Vertigo　　　　　　　　BP elevation
　　　　　　　　　　　　　　　　Slow tremors

Cardiac decompensation
↓　　　　　　　　　　　　　　　　　↓

Coronary artery disease　　　　　Central edema
　　　　　　　　　　　　　　　　　↓

Retinal hemorrhage, blurring vision, epistaxis, headache

SPECIFIC DIAGNOSES AND CARE PLANS

Risk for injury

Related to: Internal biochemica developmental regulatory function (effects of hypertension, aging)
Defining characteristics: Orthostatic hypotension, syncope, visual blurring, sustained hypertension

Outcome Criteria

Absence from trauma or injury, BP returned and maintained at baseline determinations for age and therapy.

Interventions	Rationales
Assess gradual changes in vision that includes blurring, vision loss	Decreased blood flow to retina in long term hypertension results in impaired visual acuity
Assess for dizziness, faintness when changing position (lying to upright), changes in BP in lying, sitting or standing positions at 2-3 min intervals for 15 min periods	Abrupt drop in BP occurs with quick changes to standing position as blood pools in lower part of body, cardiac output decreases and blood flow to brain is reduced; as blood volume falls, BP falls. Condition common with age and decreased baroreceptor sensing activity
Assess mental function and memory impairment	As blood flow to brain decreases, mentation is affected and compliance in medication (antihypertensives) is affected resulting in over or under medication and BP instability

Interventions	Rationales
Administer antihypertensives and adjunct medications accurately as prescribed	Lowers and regulates BP gradually and safely
Maintain clear pathways, proper lighting, articles within reach or orient to placement, walking aids such as cane, walker	Prevents trauma from bumping into furniture, falls from reaching or lack of hand rails or walking aids
Assist with ADL as needed if vision impaired	Provides care that client is unable to perform until modifications made for self-care
Assist to change positions slowly to standing, check BP and allow to stand for 3-4 min	Prevents orthostatic hypotension causing weakness and dizziness in elderly as cerebral blood flow is affected by fall in systolic pressure

Information, Instruction, Demonstration

Interventions	Rationales
Ambulating with cane or walker	Serves as aid to promote stability when walking and prevents fall
Taking pulse and blood pressure on same arm in lying and standing position and reporting elevation of more than 170 mm Hg systolic and 100 mm Hg diastolic; maintain a log of readings	Monitors BP response to therapy and sustained norms or increases to report
When arising, roll to side of bed and slowly assume sitting position by pushing with arm on bed, sitting on edge of bed for several minutes before standing	Assists to cope with orthostatic hypotension by allowing circulatory system to adjust

Interventions	Rationales
Avoid warm or hot environment, drinking alcohol, excessive exercising, hot bath or jacuzzi	Causes excessive vasodilatation and fainting
Report excessive fluid losses from diuretic, diaphoresis	Decreases blood volume which causes weakness and fainting when standing position is assumed
Wear girdle or support hose	Prevents blood pooling in abdomen or lower extremities
Daily exercise regimen	Inactivity decreases venous tone and blood return to heart resulting in orthostatic hypotension

Discharge or Maintenance Evaluation

- No falls or injuries related to visual acuity or orthostatic hypotension
- Correct administration of antihypertensives with BP maintained at baseline determinations; use of aids such as calendar, pill box with compartments
- Symptoms of orthostatic hypotension minimal or absent when assuming standing position
- Participates in ADL and exercise regimen or rehabilitation program

Noncompliance with medical regimen

Related to: Health beliefs (refusal to modify health practices and accept medical regimen)
Defining characteristics: Inability to attain goal of stabilizing BP, failure to keep appointments, failure to progress in achievement of medical regimen

Outcome Criteria

Compliance with dietary, medication and activity regimen with achievement of desired results.

Interventions	Rationales
Assess cultural influences on health beliefs, reason for noncompliance (economic, anxiety, self-esteem)	Facilitates compliance when incorporated into teaching plan
Acknowledge perceptions regarding disease and treatment	Allows for clarification of misinformation and misperception
Provide explanations of treatments in understandable language	Promotes compliance if teaching effective
Assist to plan a treatment that is acceptable and suitable to lifestyle and beliefs	Promotes compliance if plan is realistic and includes input from client and family
Encourage to monitor own BP and weight, plan own meals, take own medications	Promotes independence, control and compliance

Information, Instruction, Demonstration

Interventions	Rationales
Assist to develop and record in log, information to report to physician or referral personnel (nutritionist)	Provides comparison needed to continue or adjust regimen
Suggest support groups for smoking cessation, weight control, fitness	Encourages and supports compliance of regimen that contributes to risk factors for heart disease

Discharge or Maintenance Evaluation

- Follows plan to control BP
- Statements revealing success of medical regimen
- Statements that will comply with maintenance program after goals achieved
- Uses resources/support systems

Knowledge deficit

Related to: Lack of information or exposure to information (disease process and risk of cardiovascular disease, dietary sodium restriction, weight loss, medication administration)
Defining characteristics: Verbalization of the problem, inaccurate follow-through of instruction, request for information

Outcome Criteria

Appropriate knowledge of medical regimen prescribed to control hypertension with gradual reduction in BP to prescribed ranges

Interventions	Rationales
Assess knowledge of causes/risk factors associated with disease and methods to control and stabilize BP	Prevents repetition of information; promotes compliance of treatments necessary to maintain stable BP
Inform of potential for cardiovascular disease of CVA, renal failure, CAD and effect to vital organs with sustained hypertension	Hypertension predisposes elderly to cardiovascular disease; physiological changes in hormonal, renal, heart function
Provide explanations and information in clear and simple language that is understandable; provide limited amounts of information over periods of time rather than large amounts at one sitting	Reduces potential for noncompliance of medical regimen related to cognitive ability to understand

Interventions	Rationales
Assist in planning low sodium, fat, cholesterol diet; reduction diet if overweight or refer to nutritionist for assistance	Assist in reducing blood pressure, fluid retention
Suggest isotonic exercise plan daily to include walking, swimming, bicycling; avoid isometric exercises such as weight lifting	Enhances weight loss and blood pressure reduction, promotes circulation
Inform of proper administration including dose, frequency, method of taking, side effects and what to report, expected results from medication	Ensures that doses are not missed or increased/decreased or discontinued as BP stabilizes
Inform to avoid over-the-counter drugs without physician consent	May interact with prescribed medications
Report headache, loss of memory, nausea, vomiting, tremor	May indicate uncontrolled BP
Make and keep follow-up appointments with physician	Necessary for monitoring of diet, exercise and medication therapy and need for adjustments

Discharge or Maintenance Evaluation

- Statements of knowledge of medication administration, side effects to report
- Plans three day menu of low sodium, caloric, fat and cholesterol meals; statements of what foods to include and what foods to avoid
- Weight within baseline parameters; weight loss of 1 lb/week until baseline attained
- Absence of drug toxicity symptoms
- I&O ratio within baseline ranges
- Daily isotonic exercises for 20-30 minutes or 3 times/week as tolerated
- Limits alcohol, caffeine intake, smoking
- Practices relaxation techniques daily and when stress present

Arterial Insufficiency

Diabetes mellitus   Aging   Hyperlipidemia   Hypercholesterol

↓   →   ↓   ↓   ↓

Mycroangiopathy   Atherosclerosis (femoral, popliteal and tibial arteries)
Macroangiopathy

↓

Occlusive arterial disease

↓   →

Infection   Ischemic changes in extremities

↓

Intermittent claudication
Chronic pain or pain at rest
Absent or weak peripheral pulses
Decreased capillary filling
Thin, dry, shiny skin or extremeties
Coldness of feet, dependent erythema of legs
Pallor on leg elevation, hair loss on legs
Thickened nails on feet

↓

Ischemic lesions

↓   ↓

Diabetic ulcers over maetatarsal   Atherosclerotic obliterans ulcers
heads, on sides of soles of feet   between toes, on tips of toes, on
                                          heels, pretibial area and
                                          lateral malleolus

↓   ↓

Well-defined area
Absence of necrotic tissue
Pale color, no bleeding

↓

Healed lesions   Gangrene
Collateral circulation   ↓

Amputation

Peripheral Vascular Disease

Conditions which involve arterial or venous insufficiency associated with age related vascular changes. Venous insufficiency in the elderly is related to varicose veins, thrombosis/thrombo-phlebitis, progressive valve destruction, venous statis ulser. Arterial insufficiency in the elderly is related to progressive occlusion from atherosclerosis (arteriosclerosis obliterans, Burger's disease, intermittent claudication).

MEDICAL CARE

Analgesics: acetaminophen (Tylenol), aspirin (Bayer) PO to treat moderate leg pain by action on CNS pathways

Peripheral vasodilators: PO to increase blood flow to extremities by relaxing smooth muscle of blood vessels

Antiplatelet agents: pentoxifylline (Trental) PO to increase RBC flexibility to ease movement through capillaries, prevent intravascular coagulation, decrease RBC and platelet aggregation or dipyridamole (Persantine) or aspirin (Bayer) PO to promote blood flow and inhibit platelet aggregation

Anticoagulants: warfarin (Coumadin) PO to treat deep vein thrombophlebitis by interfering with synthesizing coagulation factors in the liver; prevents extension of existing clot and new clots from developing

Doppler ultrasonography: Reveals blood flow velocity in various parts and in extremities

Venography: Reveals venous blood flow and vein competency, filling capacity of vein, location of clot in deep vein thrombosis

Impedence plethysmography: Reveals changes in volume and rate of blood flow, degree of obstruction, venous flow in deep veins, incompetent valves, size and dilitation of veins

Oscillometry: Measures amplitude of arterial pulse

Vein ligation and stripping: Ligation of saphenous vein and removal of affected smaller veins if venous insufficiency is not controlled

Percutaneous transluminal angioplasty: Inflated balloon catheter after insertion into the artery to dilate vessel and remove obstruction; also done with laser

Endarterectomy: Removal of plaque from affected vessels

Bypass graft: Anastomosis of synthetic or vein graft to distal and proximal parts of the affected vessel after removal of the diseased part

Amputation: Removal of leg, foot, toe if disease severe and gangrene present

Prothrombin time: Decreased in presence of abnormality and done to monitor anticoagulant therapy

Lipid panel: Reveals cholesterol, triglycerides and lipid levels (LDL, HDL)

NURSING CARE PLANS

Essential nursing diagnoses and plans associated with these conditions:

Altered tissue perfusion: peripheral (6)

Related to: Interruption of arterial flow from atherosclerosis
Defining characteristics: Intermittent claudication, absent or weak peripheral pulses, decreased capillary filling, 'chronic pain or pain at rest, sparcity of hair on legs, cold feet, dependent erythema of legs, thin, dry, shiny skin, pallor on leg elevation, thick nails on feet, ischemic lesions on extremity, gangrene

Related to: Interruption of venous flow from immobility, coagulability, venous stasis, increased venous pressure, thrombus, vein inflammation
Defining characteristics: Deformed dilated varicose veins, aching pain in legs, heaviness with prolonged standing, edema, skin discoloration, positive Homans' sign, pain and deep muscle tenderness, swelling and warmth at affected area, stasis dermatitis or ulcer

Risk for trauma (198)

Related to: Internal factors of reduced temperature and/or tactile sensation
Defining characteristics: Inability to sense pain, hot/cold to extremities, bruising/trauma of extremities, altered mobility

Risk for impaired skin integrity (246)

Related to: External factor of pressure on skin from bedrest, immobility
Defining characteristics: Redness at pressure areas

Related to: Altered circulation (arterial and venous) and tissue perfusion
Defining characteristics: Thin, dry, shiny skin of extremities; ulcerations or lesions on feet; dermatitis or ulcer on leg, pigmentation on legs

SPECIFIC DIAGNOSES AND CARE PLANS

Pain

Related to: Biological injuring agents (inflammation and impaired blood flow from thrombophlebitis)
Defining characteristics: Communication of pain descriptors; guarded, protective behavior of affected leg

Chronic pain

Related to: Chronic physical disability (intermittent claudication, impaired venous emptying)
Defining characteristics: Verbal report or observed pain for more than 6 months, altered ability to continue previous activities, physical and social withdrawal

Outcome Criteria

Reduction and control of pain.

Interventions	Rationales
Assess calf pain, swelling, heat over area, deep muscle tenderness, positive Homans' sign	Signs and symptoms of venous thrombus and inflammation; venous impairment determines amount of swelling
Assess legs for feeling of heaviness, aching pain from prolonged standing	Signs and symptoms of venous insufficiency from venous stasis and varicosities
Assess pain at rest or when ambulating, amount of activity that precipitates pain	Arterial insufficiency reduces oxygen and nutrients to tissues and pain results when these needs increase as a result of activity

Interventions	Rationales
Administer mild analgesic as needed PRN	Relieves pain that is caused by inflammation or claudication
Provide progressive daily walking regimen	Promotes collateral circulation development in presence of arterial insufficiency; prevents venous stasis pain
Suggest resting when pain occurs during walking	Prevents severe arterial insufficiency in providing oxygen and nutrients to tissue
Elevate legs, support when changing position; lower legs below heart level in arterial insufficiency	Decreases pain from venous stasis and swelling, reduced arterial circulation
Provide bed cradle over legs	Prevents pain from pressure of linens on legs
Apply warm compresses to area if appropriate	Increases blood flow to area and increases pain/ inflammation

Information, Instruction, Demonstration

Interventions	Rationales
Teach clients to elevate legs for 1 hour throughout day	Promotes pain relief by assisting in venous return
Inform to avoid prolonged standing, sitting, crossing legs	Increases venous pressure leading to feeling of heaviness and aching in legs

Interventions	Rationales
Inform to avoid wearing constrictive clothing	Decreases venous return and causes increased venous pressure and pain; decreases circulation to extremities causing pain during walking

Discharge or Maintenance Evaluation

- Statements that pain controlled by rest and analgesic
- Limits sitting or standing time to 20 minute periods
- Stops walking and rests when pain occurs
- Maintains position of legs that relieves pain; elevated for venous and below heart level for arterial insufficiencies
- Absence of ischemic skin breakdown
- Progressive headling of venous leg ulcer

Activity intolerance

Related to: Generalized weakness (aging process, fatigue, chronic illness)
Defining characteristics: Communication of fatigue or weakness, presence of circulatory problem, claudication on ambulation

Related to: Bed rest or immobility (thrombophlebitis, chronic illness)
Defining characteristics: Deconditioned status, presence of circulatory problem

Venous Insufficiency

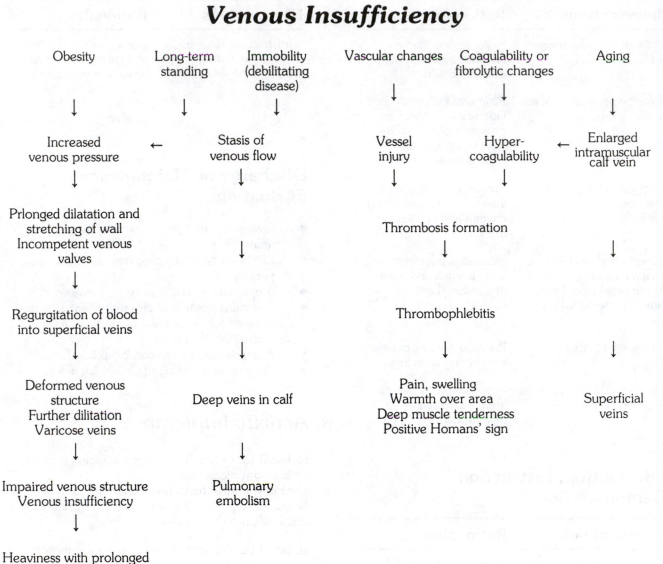

Obesity

Long-term standing

Immobility (debilitating disease)

Vascular changes

Coagulability or fibrolytic changes

Aging

Increased venous pressure ← Stasis of venous flow

Vessel injury

Hyper-coagulability ← Enlarged intramuscular calf vein

Prlonged dilatation and stretching of wall Incompetent venous valves

Thrombosis formation

Regurgitation of blood into superficial veins

Thrombophlebitis

Deformed venous structure Further dilitation Varicose veins

Deep veins in calf

Pain, swelling Warmth over area Deep muscle tenderness Positive Homans' sign

Superficial veins

Impaired venous structure Venous insufficiency

Pulmonary embolism

Heaviness with prolonged standing Aching pain in legs Skin discoloration Tissue congestion, edema Impaired tissue nutrition

Statis dermatitis Statis ulcer

Outcome Criteria

Maintained optimal activity within circulatory limitations

Interventions	Rationales
Assess baseline tolerance for activity, activity that precipitates pain, expression of fatigue, weakness	Promotes activity while protecting circulatory function
Schedule slow walk periods 2-4 times/day and stop when pain is felt	Promotes development of collateral circulation and increased activity tolerance; prevents venous stasis
Provide ROM passive or active	Immobility increases risk for venous stasis and thrombophlebitis
Apply anti-embolic hose when participating in activity	Promotes circulation during activity; prevents embolism

Information, Instruction, Demonstration

Interventions	Rationales
Walk with small steps, avoid stairways and hills, increase daily as tolerated	Provides progressive, consistent activity to improve circulation
Remove anti-embolic hose during sleep; elevate extremity	Protection of venous flow not needed during sleep to ensure venous blood flow
Suggest exercises that are comfortable and within ability and preference	Promotes compliance and satisfaction associated with success
Buerger-Allen exercises	Increases blood flow to extremities to allow for increasing activity

Discharge or Maintenance Evaluation

- Performs daily walking, rests when fatigued or before pain occurs
- Increases activity each day within scheduled limits without trauma to extremeties
- Statements that energy level and endurance increased
- Applies anti-embolic hose following a five minute elevation of affected leg before activity

Pacemaker

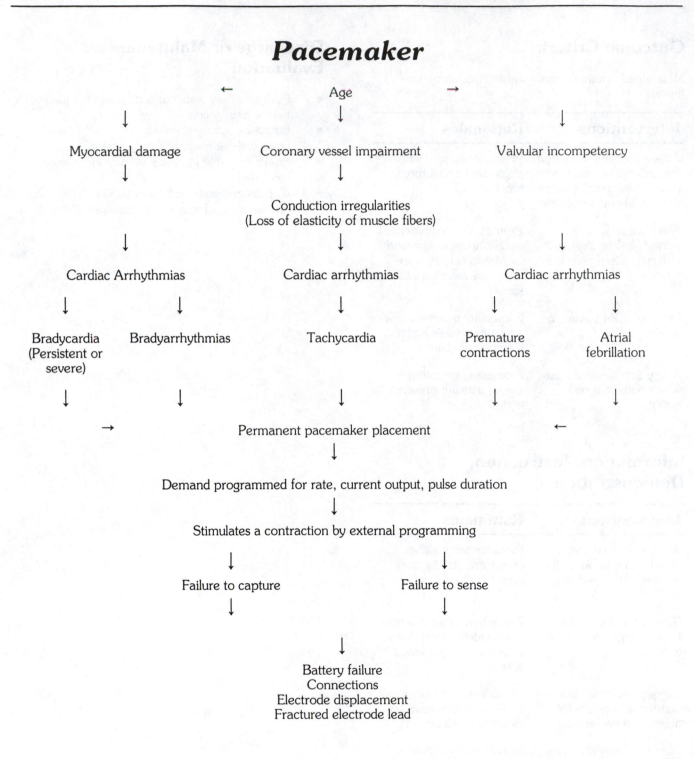

Age

Myocardial damage   Coronary vessel impairment   Valvular incompetency

Conduction irregularities
(Loss of elasticity of muscle fibers)

Cardiac Arrhythmias   Cardiac arrhythmias   Cardiac arrhythmias

Bradycardia   Bradyarrhythmias   Tachycardia   Premature   Atrial
(Persistent or   contractions   febrillation
severe)

Permanent pacemaker placement

Demand programmed for rate, current output, pulse duration

Stimulates a contraction by external programming

Failure to capture   Failure to sense

Battery failure
Connections
Electrode displacement
Fractured electrode lead

Pacemaker

A programmable electrical device consisting of a power source and a catheter electrode inserted into the right atrium, ventricle or both that provides sitmulation to the heart with conduction problems that cause a failure to provide a regular contraction. Permanent pacemakers are inserted subcutaneously in the chest or abdomen and attached to the pacing catheter placed in the heart with fluoroscopy viewing. They are indicated in the elderly for arrhythmias with or without medication therapy as heart rate decreases and conduction irregularities increase.

MEDICAL CARE

Anti-infectives: ampicillin (Amcil) PO, erythromycin (Eryc) PO to destroy microorganisms by preventing cell wall synthesis

Electrocardiography: Rhythm strips to monitor pacer function

X-ray: Confirms placement of catheter

NURSING CARE PLANS

Essential nursing diagnoses and plans associated with this condition:

Decreased cardiac output (4)

Related to: Alteration in rate, rhythm, conduction from failing batteries, break in catheter, improper pacemaker function
Defining characteristics: Variations in pulse and ECG changes

SPECIFIC DIAGNOSES AND CARE PLANS

Risk for infection

Related to: Invasive procedure (pacemaker insertion)
Defining characteristics: Redness and heat at site, pain at site, swelling and fluid collection at site

Outcome Criteria

Absence of infection at site of catheter or permanent battery.

Interventions	Rationales
Assess presence of hematoma, redness and swelling at site, temperature elevation, skin erosion	Indicates presence of infection or potential for skin breakdown
Administer antibiotic therapy; ampicillin (Amcill), erythromycin (Eryc) PO for 7 days after insertion	Prevents or treats wound infection
Empty drainage device if present	Promotes wound drainage and healing
Apply sterile dressing when needed until wound healed, avoid dislodging of catheter during site care	Maintains sterility of wound

Information, Instruction, Demonstration

Interventions	Rationales
Manifestations to observe indicating infection	Provides for measures to take and information to report for prompt treatment
How to take temperature	Monitors for potential elevation associated with infection
Clean technique to change dressing	Sterility can be maintained if proper touch technique used

Discharge or Maintenance Evaluation

- Site free of infection, intact and healed
- Statements of reportable signs indicating skin breakdown, damage or infection

Risk for injury

Related to: Internal regulatory function (pacemaker or catheter malfunction)
Defining characteristics: Arrhythmias, battery depletion or malfunction, failure of pacemaker to capture or sense, malpositioning or malfunctioning of pacing catheter

Outcome Criteria

Proper functioning and maintenance of pacemaker system with pulse rate, rhythm and duration occurring as programmed.

Interventions	Rationales
Assess pulse, changes in cardiac output, changes in ECG	Decreased pulse (5-10/min) and cardiac output indicate battery depletion; changes in ECG may indicate perforation, loss of capture, arrhythmias from irritation of ventricular wall by electrode
Troubleshoot for sensing or capture failure	Prevents pacemaker failure or corrects functional problem
Assess VS, apical-radial pulse, decreased urinary output, palpitations, chest pain, fatigue, dyspnea, lightheadedness	Signs and symptoms of pacemaker malfunction
Provide ROM to shoulder if appropriate and ordered	Prevents frozen shoulder but may aggrevate condition brought about by malposition of pacing catheter

Information, Instruction, Demonstration

Interventions	Rationales
Using manufacturers instructions, familiarize with parts, function, results expected, signs of failure to report	Provides understanding of type of and function of pacemaker
Method of taking pulse, variations and what to report	Monitors for desired effect of pacemaker
Importance of follow-up and continued visits to physician	Ensures monitoring for malfunction, battery depletion

Interventions	Rationales
Participate in activities but avoid blows to chest, contact sports	Pacemaker usually permits improved activity tolerance
Wear clothing that is loose-fitting around pacemaker	Prevents revealing presence of pacemaker and promotes body image
Avoid microwave ovens, other electrical interference; request hand scanner at airports	Some pacemakers are still affected by electrical interference or current leakage
Send rhythm strips when requested	Permits monitoring of heart activity and pacemaker function
Carry identification card or wear bracelet with pacemaker type, model, physician, site of insertion	Provides information for emergency care

Discharge or Maintenance Evaluation

- Wears or carrys proper identification information
- Reports to and visits physician as recommended
- Checks pulse daily; states acceptable variations in pulse
- Properly grounds all electrical equipment for safe environment; avoids exposure to electrical interferences if necessary
- Provides transtelephone rhythm strips periodically as directed
- Reviews manufacturers instruction guide; statements of signs to report
- Maintains special diet if prescribed, activity schedule to include exercise, sex, occupation, travel, other
- Procedure for changing battery in the hospital if and when needed
- Limits manipulation to prevent dislodging of catheter

Respiratory System

Respiratory System

Pulmonary changes in the geriatric client occur at different rates for different individuals with the most pronounced changes occurring over 70 years of age. The general physical health and conditioning as one ages affect the efficiency of respiratory function. Pulmonary parameters of the aging lungs depend on changes in lung structure and function, gas exchange and pulmonary circulation, homeostasis and ventilatory control which increase the work of breathing. Age imposes limitations on the respiratory system that become evident on exertion or stress as the aging client uses more energy to expand the chest, an important activity in carrying out respiratory function, and suffers a reduced functional reserve, an important factor in creating an increased vulnerability to respiratory infections and diseases. Changes due to aging and environmental effects on lungs are continuous and long term causing some degree of reduced ventilation and altered ventilation/perfusion. Lung cancer is the most common neoplasm associated with the respiratory system in the elderly population.

GENERAL RESPIRATORY CHANGES ASSOCIATED WITH THE AGING PROCESS

Chest structure and bronchopulmonary movement

- Increased stiffness and rigidity of fibrous connective tissue, lymphoid elements and muscles causing reduced bronchopulmonary movement, decreased strength of muscles used in breathing, increased use of accessory muscles and. diaphragm for breathing.
- Increased stiffness and rigidity of rib cage causing reduced rib mobility and ability for chest expansion.
- Calcification of cartilage at rib articulation areas causing decreased expansion (compliance) of chest wall.
- Increased anteroposterior chest diameter in relation to lateral diameter (barrel chest). This normally results in no particular changes in chest movement unless kyphosis and/or dorsal scoliosis is present, causing stooped posture which affects localized lung expansion and change in spinal curvature in the lumbar region.
- Reduced reflex activity of coughing and ciliary movement caused by decreased muscle tone and strength, decreased sensitivity to stimuli, and drying and atrophy of mucous membranes causing decreased cough ability and bronchoelimination.

Breathing pattern and ventilatory function

- Shallow and more rapid respiratory rate causing decreased amount of air taken in.
- Restriction in pulmonary expansion and contraction or obstruction of pulmonary airways by mucus causing reduced ventilatory function.
- Loss of lung elasticity, compliance and air retained in lung bases (increased pressure in alveoli during inspiration) after expiration causing decreased vital capacity (maximal volume of air expired after a maximal inspiration) and increased residual air (volume of air remaining in lungs after a maximal expiration).
- Reduced respiratory excursion causing difficulty in breathing deeply or holding breath when asked to do so.
- Increased respiratory rate caused by anxiety or exertion accentuated by reduced energy reserve and weakness; uncoordinated pattern in rate and depth or a disruption in usual pattern caused by exertion or a chronic respiratory condition.
- Increased weakness of chest muscles causing impaired respiratory efficiency.

Lung and respiratory gas exchange function

- Changes in the properties and distribution of elastin and collagen causing loss of lung and blood vessel elasticity and change in the volume pressure of the lungs as a result of impaired elasticity and reduced mobility of chest cage.
- Decreased elasticity, expansibility of areas (rigid lungs) and obstruction to air flow in areas causing decreased distribution of air to functioning alveoli and alteration in intrapulmonary mixing.
- Decreased number of alveoli, loss of lung capillaries, decreased respiratory rate, decreased oxygen saturation (5% decrease attributed to aging process) and expired carbon dioxide causing decreased gas exchange.
- Decreased force of lung recoil as lung elasticity decreases causing collapse of smaller bronchiole.
- Under ventilation of lower lung fields causing poor aeration of bases and reduced distribution of air to functioning and well perfused alveoli; increased apical ventilation causing decreased PaO_2.
- Progressive hyperventilation with decreased vital capacity and increased residual air as lung elasticity is lost causing slight hyperresonance on percussion and decreased or slightly quieter breath sounds on auscultation
- Hydrogen ion concentration more easily disturbed with slowed return to normal levels causing greater potential for acid-base imbalance.
- Reduced rate of movement of gases across alveolocapillary membrane and thickened alveolocapillary membrane causing greater potential for impaired gas exchange.

ESSENTIAL NURSING DIAGNOSES AND CARE PLANS

Ineffective airway clearance

Related to: Decreased energy and fatigue
Defining characteristics: Changes in rate, depth of respirations, tachypnea

Related to: Tracheobronchial infection, obstruction, secretion
Defining characteristics: Abnormal breath sounds (crackles, wheezes), changes in rate, depth of respirations; tachypnea, dyspnea, ineffective or effective cough with or without sputum, cyanosis

Outcome Criteria

Return to or maintenance of respiratory baselines with patent airways.

Interventions	Rationales
Assess energy level and endurance and effect on chest expansion	Decreases with age; more than one chronic disorder (present in 4 out 5 of elderly) further compromises maintenance of ventilation
Assess respiratory status for rate, depth and ease, essence of tachypnea, dyspnea in relation to disease process or decreased energy level	Changes vary from minimal to extreme caused by obstruction (bronchial swelling), increased mucus secretions (over-secretions of goblet cells, tracheobronchial infection), bronchospasm and narrowing of air passages (stimulation of irritant receptors in smooth muscle layer of conducting airways)

Interventions	Rationales
Auscultate for adventitious sounds (crackles, wheezes)	Wheezes result from squeezing of air past narrowed airways during expiration caused by bronchospasms, edema and obstructive secretions; crackles result from lung consolidation of leukocytes and fibrin in an area caused by infectious process or fluid accumulation in the lungs
Assess for cyanosis	Not a reliable indicator of loss of airway patency as it does not occur until a level of 5 g of reduced Hb/100ml blood in superficial capillaries is reached which occurs late in chronic respiratory disease
Assess cough and sputum production for amount, color, viscosity, ability to cough and expectorate secretions in relation to energy level	Changes in color to green in morning and to yellow during day indicate infection; tenacious, thick secretions require more energy and effort to remove and may cause obstruction and stasis leading to infection and respiratory changes
Administer bronchodilators, anti-inflammatories, expectorants, mucolytics, anti-infectives PO, SC, by hand-held inhaler device, small volume nebulizer, IPPB	Treats bronchospasms, prevents or treats infection, liquifies secretions and enhances outflow and removal of respiratory tract fluids
Provide environmental air humidification	Adds moisture to the air to thin mucus for easier removal
Offer 2-3 L (10-12 glasses)/day unless contraindicated; offer hourly including a warm beverage upon arising	Assists to mobilize and thin secretions for easier removal

Interventions	Rationales
Position in semi-Fowler's and change position q2h	Prevents accumulation of secretions; promotes comfort and ease of breathing and decreases airflow resistance and enhances gas distribution; facilitates chest expansion
Perform postural drainage using gravity, percussion, vibration; avoid positions that may be contraindicated in the elderly	Raises secretions, clears sputum and increases force of expiration
Maintain activity pattern, encourage ambulation within limitations	Mobilizes secretions for easier removal
Encourage deep breathing and coughing exercises by taking a deep breath, exhale as much as possible, inhale again and cough forcefully twice from chest	Assists in dislodging secretions for easier expectoration by initiating the cough reflex which protects the lungs from accumulation of secretions by action on receptors in the tracheobronchial wall
Suction if appropriate	Removes secretions in those too weak to cough or with mentation or LOC deficits

Information, Instruction, Demonstration

Interventions	Rationales
Avoid milk, caffeine drinks, alcohol	Milk thickens mucus, caffeine reduces effect of medications (bronchodilators), alcohol increases cell dehydration and bronchial constriction

Interventions	Rationales
Avoid excessively hot or cold fluids; cold air and wind exposure by wearing mask	Predisposes to coughing spells; dyspnea, bronchospasm
Encourage cessation of smoking; suggest program to support the reduction or cessation of smoking	Smoking causes increased mucus, vasoconstriction, increased BP, inflammation of lung lining, decreased number of macrophages in airways and mucociliary blanket
Program of daily exercises; supervise if needed	Promotes secretion removal
Avoid crowds and those with upper respiratory infections	Prevents possible transmission of infection
Proper use of and disposal of tissues used for expectoration	Prevents transmission of microorganisms as sputum contains infecting organisms and inflammatory debris
Use of hand-held inhaler, small volume nebulizer, administration of oral medications, nose drops	Promotes correct administration of medication for optimal effect

Discharge or Maintenance Evaluation

- Breath sounds clear with optimal air flow; rate, depth and ease within baseline determinations.
- Ability to cough up secretions that are thin and clear following deep breathing/coughing exercises.
- Effective daily bronchoelimination resulting in patent airways.
- Bronchodilators, expectorants, mucolytics effective in preventing bronchospasms, thick secretions that cling to wall of airway system, difficulty in removal of secretions.

Ineffective breathing pattern

Related to: Pain
Defining characteristics: Respiratory depth changes

Related to: Anxiety
Defining characteristics: Dyspnea

Related to: Imflammatory process
Defining characteristics: Tachypnea, cough, decreased fremitus, crackles

Related to: Decreased lung expansion
Defining characteristics: Dyspnea, respiratory depth changes, increased anteroposterior diameter, altered chest excursion, decreased energy and fatigue

Related to: Tracheobronchial obstruction
Defining characteristics: Tachypnea, dyspnea, cough, use of accessory muscles, respiratory depth changes, pursed-lip breathing/prolonged expiratory phase, assumption of a three.point position, abnormal arterial blood gases

Outcome Criteria

Return to or maintenance of respiratory baselines with breathing pattern at optimal level within energy and disease parameters.

Interventions	Rationales
Assess respiratory status for rate, depth and ease, presence of dyspnea and use of accessory muscles, lengthened expiratory phase, palpate for chest configuration	Changes vary with acuteness of condition and are caused by airway resistance, bronchospasms, decreased lung expansion; dyspnea results from stimulation of lung receptors or reduced ventilatory capacity or breathing reserve
Assess energy level, fatigue and effect on breathing	Limited energy reserve in elderly quickly dissipated as work of breathing increases

Interventions	Rationales
Pain or chest discomfort, sore chest muscles, effect on chest excursion	Results from excessive coughing, use of muscles for work of breathing causing reduced chest expansion and shallow breathing pattern
Auscultate for diminished or absent breath sounds, wheezes or crackles, percuss for hyperresonance, increased tactile fremitus	Changes caused by infectious process as consolidation develops; damage to bronchioles restricts air movement
Administer broncho-dilators; use sedatives or tranquilizers judiciously; anti-infectives PO	Treats bronchospasms, prevents or treats infection, respiratory efficiency reduced by sedatives and tranquilizers but may be given to promote rest and reduce anxiety
Position in semi- or high-Fowler's or orthopneic using an overbed table and pillow	Promotes comfort and ease of breathing and gas distribution; facilitates chest expansion by causing abdominal organs to sag away from diaphragm
Perform deep breathing exercises and pursed-lip breathing; isometric exercises for intercostal muscles and diaphragm strengthening; upper body exercises by raising arms and using 2-3 lb hand weights if able	Strengthens chest and abdominal muscles to enhance breathing; pursed-lip breathing prolongs expiratory phase and prevents alveoli from collapsing to decrease CO_2 retention
Provide proper body alignment in positioning for sleep, use pillows, foam rubber wedge to elevate head and support chest	Ensures optimal ventilation; supine position reduces total lung capacity by 300 ml
Pace activities, allow for rest between periods of exercises	Prevents changes in respirations brought about by exertion

Information, Instruction, Demonstration

Interventions	Rationales
Avoid extending any activity beyond baseline of tolerance	Causes exacerbation of dyspnea
Gradually increase activities and exercises as endurance increases based on pulmonary stress test	Increases energy and participation in ADL
Relaxation techniques: guided imagery, music when breathing pattern changes or anxiety increases	Decreases respiratory rate
Avoid over-the-counter drugs unless approved by a physician	May cause drug interactions with prescribed medications
Environment with optimal temperature, humidity, ventilation, free of allergens	Removes irritants that affect breathing

Discharge or Maintenance Evaluation

- Breath sounds clear with respiratory rate, depth and ease within baseline determinations.
- Absence of dyspnea with breathing effort maintained at baseline determination.
- Improved chest expansion resulting from exercise program.
- Decreased airway resistance following administration of bronchodilators; improved breathing following rest and relaxation, administration of sedatives.

Impaired gas exchange

Related to: Ventilation perfusion imbalance

Defining characteristics: Confusion, somnolence, restlessness, irritability, inability to move secretions, hypercapnea, hypoxia

Outcome Criteria

Maintenance of adequate oxygen and carbon dioxide levels with return of respiratory baselines.

Interventions	Rationales
Assess respiratory status for rate, depth and ease, dyspnea and respiratory effort on exertion, length of inspiratory versus expiratory phase	Gas exchange carried out by pulmonary circulation is affected by body position and posture as is ventilation; it is dependent on the matching of ventilation and perfusion of equal amounts of air and blood entering the lungs at the alveoli level. Changes in respiratory pattern or airways may result in gas exchange disturbances
Assess for cyanosis and monitor arterial blood gases for decreased O_2 and increased CO_2 levels, possible lowered pH; O_2 saturation by oximetry	O_2 and CO_2 diffusion and exchange are affected by the surface area available, thickness of the alveolocapillary membrane both of which are characteristic of aging or diseased lung tissue; cyanosis results from the reduction in oxygenated hemoglobin in the blood and leads to hypoxia (reduced tissue oxygenation)
Assess for changes in consciousness, mentation, restlessness, irritability, rapid fatigue	Results of decreased oxygen to brain tissue with progressive hypoxia
Position in semi- or high-Fowler's using chair or pillow on overbed table to lean forward	Promotes breathing and gas distribution; facilitates chest expansion and pulmonary blood flow; sitting position stabilizes chest structures

Interventions	Rationales
Breathing exercises and retraining	Restores function of diaphragm which decreases work of breathing and improves gas exchange
Administer oxygen at 2-3 L/min via cannula, non-breather mask or Venturi mask	Maintains adequate oxygen level without depressing respiratory drive which increases CO_2 retention; 4-8 L/min if COPD not present
Provide for early recognition of impending hypoxia and effects on nervous system (mental clouding), circulatory system (tachycardia), respiratory system (dyspnea), gastronintestinal system (nausea, vomiting)	Hypoxia considered mild until O_2 level falls below 60 mm Hg and severe when O_2 level falls to 40-50 mm Hg

Information, Instruction, Demonstration

Interventions	Rationales
Avoid activities that cause change in respirations especially shortness of breath	Increase in oxygen consumption changes breathing pattern
Application of cannula; administering oxygen by compressed air in a cylinder, liquid oxygen system or oxygen concentrator	Methods of oxygen administration vary in cost and portability
Correct amount of oxygen to administer	Ensures appropriate amounts to prevent hypoxia

Interventions	Rationales
Report any changes in fatigue level or any mental clouding, increasing dyspneic episodes	Indicates impending hypoxia
Cautions with use of oxygen (no open flames, smoking, use of greasy products) and post signs	Safe environment as oxygen supports combustion

Discharge or Maintenance Evaluation

- Respiratory rate, depth and ease within baseline determinations.
- ABGs with O_2, CO_2, pH and O_2 saturation within normal ranges with allowances made for changes resulting from aging process.
- Adequate oxygenation of tissues (absence of hypoxia), with correct adminstration of oxygen, continuous or PRN before and after activity, during sleep.
- Assumes most comfortable and effective position for optimal chest expansion and ventilation.
- Environment safe for O_2 administration

Asthma

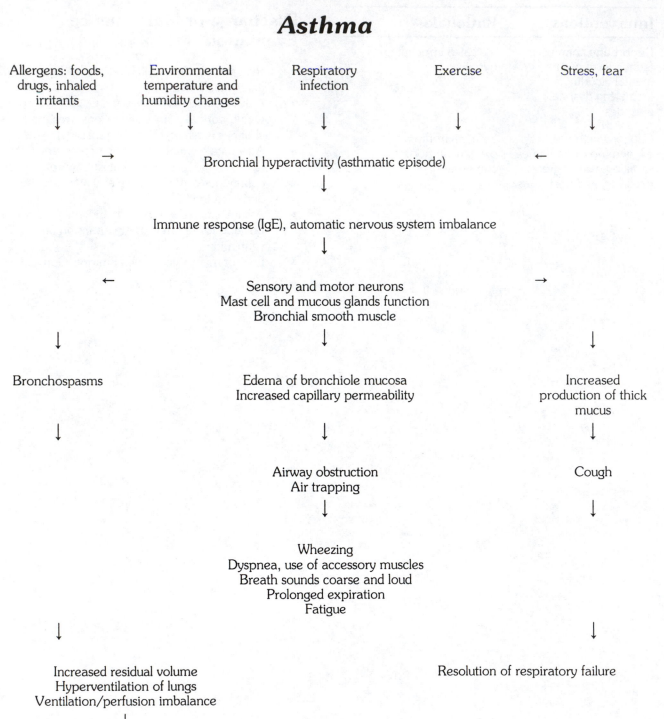

Allergens: foods, drugs, inhaled irritants → Environmental temperature and humidity changes → Respiratory infection → Exercise ← Stress, fear

Bronchial hyperactivity (asthmatic episode)

Immune response (IgE), automatic nervous system imbalance

Sensory and motor neurons
Mast cell and mucous glands function
Bronchial smooth muscle

Bronchospasms

Edema of bronchiole mucosa
Increased capillary permeability

Increased production of thick mucus

Airway obstruction
Air trapping

Cough

Wheezing
Dyspnea, use of accessory muscles
Breath sounds coarse and loud
Prolonged expiration
Fatigue

Increased residual volume
Hyperventilation of lungs
Ventilation/perfusion imbalance

Resolution of respiratory failure

Cyanosis

Chronic Obstructive Pulmonary Disease

Chronic pulmonary conditions affect the function of the pulmonary system by creating airway obstruction which results in a reduction of air movement in and out of the lungs. COPD is the most common cause of pulmonary disability in the aged population and includes asthma, emphysema and chronic bronchitis. Many elderly are found to have both chronic bronchitis and emphysema concurrently. Changes in the respiratory system such as loss of elasticity, decreased vital capicity and increased residual air associated with aging contribute to the progressive severity of these diseases.

MEDICAL CARE

Bronchodilators: theophylline (Slo-Bid, Theo-Dur) PO or aminophylline (theophylline ethylenediamine) IV to produce bronchodilation by relaxing bronchial smooth muscle; **adrenergics:** epinephrine (Adrenalin) SC, albuterol (Ventolin), isoproterenol (Isuprel), isoetharine (Bronkosol) by inhalation to relax bronchial smooth muscle; **anticholinergics:** ipratropium bromide (Atrovent) by inhalation to relax larger central airways

Antiasthmatics: cromolyn sodium (Intal) by inhalation to prevent allergic reactions by stabilizing the mast cells and preventing release of the inflammatory mediators which cause an asthmatic attack

Expectorants: guaifenesin with codeine PO to stimulate bronchial secretory cells to increase production of respiratory tract secretions, guaifenesin (Robitussin) PO to irritate gastric mucosa to stimulate gastric reflex and production of respiratory secretions

Mucolytics: acetylcysteine (Mucomyst) by inhalation to liquefy thick, tenacious mucus for easier removal, guaifenesin (Humibid) PO to liquefy thick mucus for easier mobilization and removal by coughing

Corticosteroids: prednisone (Deltasone) PO, flunisolide (Aero-Bid) by inhalation as anti-inflammatory to bolster body defenses when exposed to potential infection, allergic reaction

Anti-infectives: ampicillin (Amcil), cefuroxine (Ceftin), erythromycin (Eryc) PO to treat infections by inhibiting cell wall synthesis

Oxygen therapy: Treats hypoxemia as indicated by ABGs, oximetry

Chest x-ray: Reveals hyperinflation, flattened diaphragm in those with asthma, emphysema; thickened bronchial walls and possible right ventricular hypertrophy in those with chronic bronchitis

Pulmonary function: Reveals increased total lung capacity, residual volume, decreased forced vital capacity, expiratory and forced flow rate

Sputum culture: Identifies airway or lung infections and sensitivity to specific antibiotics

Arterial blood gasses: Reveals decrease in O_2 and later increase in CO_2 levels as disease progresses; decrease in pH with impending acidosis

CBC: Increase in WBC if infection is present; increase in RBC as body compensates for increased need for oxygen transport to tissues

Theophylline level: Reveals need for drug adjustment for optimal effect or to prevent toxicity

Chronic Bronchitis

Smoking   Recurrent respiratory infections   Inhaled substances

↓   ↓   ↓

Inflammation of bronchial glands, edema of bronchial glands,   Overproduction of mucus
Hyperplasia of bronchial glands

↓   ↓   ↓

Airway obstruction of large and small airways   ←   ↓
Increased airway resistance

Progressive chronic
production cough

↓   ↓

Dyspnea   Pulmonary hypertension
Ventilation/perfusion imbalance   Right heart failure or cor pulmonale

↓   ↓

Chronic hypoxemia and hypercapnia   Peripheral edema
Clubbing of fingers

↓   Dyspnea at rest
Expiratory crackles and wheezes

Cyanosis
Polycythemia

NURSING CARE PLANS

Essential nursing diagnoses and plans associated with these conditions:

Ineffective airway clearance (44)

Related to: Decreased energy and fatigue from work of breathing
Defining characteristics: Inability to cough and raise secretions, tachypnea, fatigue

Related to: Tracheobronchial infection, obstruction, secretion
Defining characteristics: Bronchospasms, ineffective cough, stasis of secretions, crackles/wheezes, changes in rate, depth of respirations, increased production of mucus

Ineffective breathing pattern (45)

Related to: Anxiety and fear of suffocation
Defining characteristics: Dyspnea, shortness of breath

Related to: Pain and sore muscles of chest
Defining characteristics: Excessive coughing and use of accessory muscles

Related to: Decreased lung expansion and hyperinflation
Defining characteristics: Respiratory depth changes, dyspnea, increased anteroposterior diameter

Related to: Tracheobronchial obstruction
Defining characteristics: Cough, dyspnea, use of accessory muscles, abnormal ABGs, prolonged expiratory phase, respiratory depth changes, excessive mucus production

Impaired gas exchange (47)

Related to: Ventilation perfusion imbalance
Defining characteristics: Mental cloudiness, confusion, hypoxemia, hypercapnea (ABGs), cyanosis

Altered nutrition: less than body requirements (118)

Related to: Inability to ingest food from biologic factors
Defining characteristics: Loss of weight, weakness, difficulty in mastication, swallowing with dyspnea (air swallowing), fatigue from effort in breathing, nausea and anorexia from medication; inflammed, sore buccal cavity from inhaled corticosteroids

Sleep pattern disturbance (77)

Related to: Internal factors of illness and psychological stress of dyspnea
Defining characteristics: Interrupted sleep, irritability, not feeling well rested

Sexual dysfunction (181)

Related to: Altered body function caused by disease process
Defining characteristics: Dyspnea on exertion, fatigue, limitations imposed by disease, alteration in achieving desired satisfaction

SPECIFIC DIAGNOSES AND CARE PLANS

Anxiety

Related to: Threat of death (severe bronchospasm and dyspnea)
Defining characteristics: Communication of apprehension, fear, feeling of suffocation and uncertain outcome

Related to: Change in health status (chronic, pregressive nature of disease and effect on lifestyle)
Defining characteristics: Communication of increased helplessness and feelings of inadequacy

Emphysema

Smoking   Environmental   Repeated   Alpha 1-   Aging
                 pollution   respiratory   antitrypsin   process
                                        infections   deficiency

   ↓   ↓   ↓   ↓   ↓

                                                                           ←

Loss of elastin from alveoli and airways
Enlargement and destruction of air spaces distal or terminal   Changes in thoracic spine
bronchioles   Enlarged thorax
Sclerotic changes

↓   ↓

Loss of alveolar tissue   Stretching and overdistention
Loss of alveolar diffusing surface   of peripheral alveoli
Loss of compliance and elasticity

↓   ↓

Air trapping in alveoli   Breakdown of walls
Increased airway size on inspiration   of alveoli
Collapse of small airways on expiration
Hyperinflation of lungs

↓   ↓

Dyspnea, use of accessory muscles of alveoli   Postural or senile
Barrel chest appearance   emphysema
Prolonged expiratory phase
Decreased breath sounds
Fatigue
Weight loss

↓

Progressive deterioration from dyspnea on
exertion to dyspnea at rest

↓

Respiratory failure

Outcome Criteria

Reduced or manageable anxiety level.

Interventions	Rationales
Assess changes in anxiety level during periods of dyspnea; feelings of helplessness, fear of suffocation or death	Anxiety may reach panic level during severe dyspnea, exertional dyspnea creates anxiety reflective of severity of dyspnea and disabilities resulting from it
Provide calm, supportive environment during dyspnea	Reduces anxiety which will increase dyspnea if not brought under control
Speak slowly and quietly with slow, regular pattern to breathing	Assists in slowing breathing
Provide relaxation exercises, guided imagery, autogenic technique	Reduces anxiety by distraction and slows breathing

Information, Instruction, Demonstration

Interventions	Rationales
Value of psychotherapy in learning to use relaxation, diversionary techniques to reduce anxiety	Provides wider range of techniques to reduce anxiety
Potential for depressed respirations if taking sedatives, antianxiety agents	Acts on respiratory center to depress respirations

Discharge or Maintenance Evaluation

- Dyspneic episode and associated anxiety relieved or decreased.

- Communication that exertional dyspnea and associated anxiety controlled as activity intolerance avoided.

Activity intolerance

Related to: Generalized weakness (fatigue, inadequate sleep, work of breathing)
Defining characteristics: Communication of weakness, feeling tired, dyspnea, increased pulse and blood pressure during activity

Related to: Imbalance between oxygen supply and demand (hypoxia)
Defining characteristics: Dyspnea, reduced oxygen saturation level

Outcome Criteria

Maintenance of optimal activity level within energy and breathing limitations.

Interventions	Rationales
Assess for baseline tolerance for activity, ability to adapt, amount of rest and sleep	Promotes and protects respiratory functions
Assess pulse and respirations before, during and after activity	Pulse increase of 10 or more/min or increase and any difficulty in respirations indicate that activity limit has been reached
Provide periods of rest after activity; schedule activities around rest or sleep periods; allow self-pacing of activities	Prevents dyspneic episode and provides uninterrupted rest and sleep necessary for physical and mental health to prevent fatigue
Quiet, stress-free environment	Stress and stimuli produce anxiety and increase respirations

Interventions	Rationales
Provide oxygen during activities if appropriate	Pulmonary function tests indicate hypoxemia during exercise and determine need for additional oxygen
Assist with activities as needed	Conserves energy and oxygen consumption; prevents dyspnea
Provide slowly progressive activity/exercise program and promote independent ADL participation	Increases delivery of oxygen to tissues; increases tolerance to activities and decreases feelings of helplessness

Information, Instruction, Demonstration

Interventions	Rationales
Avoid extending activities beyond fatigue level or tolerance that may provoke dyspnea	Conserves energy and prevents exacerbation of dyspnea
Utilize energy saving devices such as arm rests, sitting on stool in shower, placing articles commonly used within reach; simplification strategies depending on severity of impairment	Prevents fatigue
Consider pulmonary rehabilitation program and continue prescribed regimen on a daily basis	Increases energy level and endurance, muscle strength
Schedule activities during peak or optimal effect time of systemic medications; use inhalers before activity	Allows for activities without dyspneic episode

Interventions	Rationales
Inform of inspiration and expiration pattern when performing a task; contact American Lung Association for breathing techniques during activities	Allows for more effective breathing during activity

Discharge or Maintenance Evaluation

- Activity tolerance within baseline determinations
- Minimal dyspnea and absence of hypoxia during activities
- Correct administration of bronchodilators in relation to activities
- Increased energy and endurance with progressive self-care in ADL
- Daily follow-through of exercise regimen

Risk for infection

Related to: Inadequate primary defenses (decrease in ciliary action, stasis of body fluids)
Defining characteristics: Depression of cough reflex or inability to cough up secretions, impaired mucociliary blanket, reduced pulmonary macrophages

Related to: Chronic disease (COPD)
Defining characteristics: Loss of respiratory defense mechanisms over long term, impairment of their effectiveness

Outcome Criteria

Absence of upper or lower respiratory infection.

Interventions	Rationales
Assess for increased dyspnea, change in color and viscosity of sputum (yellow or green), cough, low grade temperature	Early detection of respiratory infection allows for immediate treatment before respiratory system is compromised

Interventions	Rationales
Administer antibiotic therapy	Prevents or treats respiratory infection if symptoms appear
Obtain periodic sputum cultures	Reveals infectious agent, evaluates effect of treatment

Information, Instruction, Demonstration

Interventions	Rationales
Avoid smoking, chilling, inhalation of environmental pollutants	Irritates mucosa and initiates dyspneic attack
Avoid large groups, exposure to those with URI	Prevents contact with potential infectious agents
Proper handwashing, disposal of tissues, cover mouth and nose when coughing, cleansing and disinfection of respiratory equipment	Prevents transmission of infectious agents from contaminated articles
Proper administration and expected effect of antibiotic therapy and to take complete prescription	Prevent recurrence of infection
Advise to have flu and pneumonia immunization	Those with COPD highly susceptible to infections
Report fever or change in sputum	Indicates infection
Regular change of air conditioner filters	Removes pollutants from air

Discharge or Maintenance Evaluation

- Temperature within normal range, sputum clear
- Ability to cough and remove secretions

- Immunization for pneumonia, yearly influenza immunization obtained
- Daily disinfection of respiratory equipment and handwashing when appropriate

Ineffective individual coping

Related to: Multiple life changes (limitations imposed on life style by COPD)
Defining characteristics: Inability to meet role expectations, inability to meet basic needs, alteration in societal participation, chronic fatigue, chronic worry

Related to: Inadequate coping method
Defining characteristics: Inability to problem solve, inappropriate use of defense mechanisms, poor self-esteem, chronic anxiety

Outcome Criteria

Adaption to chronic, disabling disease with optimal adjustments in lifestyle in relation to respiratory function.

Interventions	Rationales
Assess use of coping skills, ability to cope with fear associated with changes in breathing pattern and fatigue, chronicity of worry and anxiety	Older adults display outstanding ability to cope and adapt, although inability to maintain independence and control over life leads to frustration and negative feelings about lifestyle
Assist to identify positive defense mechanisms and promote their use; new behaviors to be learned	Use of defense mechanisms that have worked in past increases ability to cope and promotes self-esteem
Provide environment that allows for free expression of concerns and fears	Encourages trust and relieves anxiety

Information, Instruction, Demonstration

Interventions	Rationales
Social and coping skills with problem solving approaches	Prevents disengagement and promotes coping ability with lifestyle changes
Relaxation techniques	Reduces anxiety and stress associated with decreasing respiratory function
New ways or methods to adapt roles to new situation or needs	Provides for alternatives that increase participation and independence in activities
Suggest psychotherapy or support groups if appropriate	Provides variety of techniques to reduce anxiety and stress

Discharge or Maintenance Evaluation

- Uses appropriate coping and problem-solving skills in adapting to functional losses
- Level of independence appropriate for functional ability
- Asks for assistance when needed
- Verbalization of reduced anxiety and fear
- Participation in social activities according to preference and activity tolerance

Influenza

An acute inflammation of the nasopharynx, trachea and bronchioles with associated edema, congestion and possible necrosis of these respiratory structures. The highest priority risk group includes those over 65 years of age, those with chronic cardiovascular or pulmonary diseases and residents of long term, chronic care facilities. Several different strains of the virus cause the disease and new strains appear which results in yearly changes in immunization precautions for the elderly.

MEDICAL CARE

Analgesics, antipyretics: acetaminophen (Tylenol), aspirin (Ecotrin, Bayer) PO to reduce temperature by action on the hypothalamus control center, treat headache, general aches and pain by action on CNS pathways

Antivirals: amatadine HCl (Symmetrel) PO to inhibit virus shedding or for prophylaxis after exposure to disease

Nose drops: phenyephrine (Neo-synephrine 0.25%) to relieve nasal congestion

Flu vaccine: Injection to provide immunity to prevent disease in those at risk

Chest x-ray: To reveal possible lung involvement or complications

Sputum culture: To identify viral lung infection/pneumonia; sensitivities to reveal specific antibiotic effect on organism

NURSING CARE PLANS

Essential nursing diagnoses and plans associated with this condition:

Ineffective airway clearance (44)

Related to: Tracheobronchial and nasal secretions
Defining characteristics: Rhinorrhea, irritating unproductive cough, change in rate and depth of respirations

Ineffective breathing pattern (45)

Related to: Inflammatory process from viral infection
Defining characteristics: Tachypnea, cough

SPECIFIC DIAGNOSES AND CARE PLANS

Pain

Related to: Biological injuring agent (influenza virus)
Defining characteristics: Communication of pain descriptors, autonomic responses

Outcome Criteria

Relief or absence of pain.

Interventions	Rationales
Assess headache, sore throat, redness of throat, general malaise, muscle aches and pain	Result of inflammation, elevated temperature
Assess Herpes simplex lesions on lips or mouth	Associated with viral infection
Assess VS for increased R, BP and P changes from baselines; usually increased	Result of autonomic response to pain

Influenza

Airborne droplets   Direct contact with infected person
↓   ↓

Myxovirus inflenzae
Type A, B, C
↓

Susceptible cells/host
↓

Replication and spread to other cells
↓

↓   ↓   ↓

Inflammation of   Desquamation of   Destruction of cilia of
upper airway   upper airway   upper airway
↓

Chills, fever, malaise
Sore throat, cough
Sneezing, profile nasal discharge
Headache, anorexia

↓   ↓   ↓

Viral pneumonia   Resolution
COPD exacerbation
Death

Interventions	Rationales
Administer mild analgesic	Controls aches and pains by inhibiting brain prostaglandin synthesis
Provide restful, quiet environment	Reduces stimuli that increases pain
Provide warm baths or heating pad to aching muscles, watch for orthostatic changes	Warmth causes vasodilation and decreases discomfort
Provide cool compress to head	Promotes comfort and treats headache
Provide backrub	Promotes relaxation and relieves aches
Encourage gargling with warm water, provide throat lozenges	Reduces throat discomfort

Discharge or Maintenance Evaluation

- Analgesic is effective in reducing pain and discomfort
- Client verbalizes relief from headache, sore throat, and muscle pains
- Vital signs returned to baselines

Hyperthermia

Related to: Illness (influenza)
Defining characteristics: Increase in body temperature above normal range

Outcome Criteria

Temperature reduced to baseline level.

Interventions	Rationales
Assess temperature for elevation, presence of chills, diaphoresis, dry, flushed skin that is warm to touch	Elevated temperature is response to inflammatory process associated with influenza
Administer antipyretic	Prevents extreme elevations to protect vulnerable body organs such as the brain
Provide sponge baths	Increases heat loss by evaporation
Cooling mattress if appropriate	Removes heat by conduction into the cool solution that circulates in the mattress
Provide fluid intake of up to 3 L/day (10-12 glasses)	Supports hypermetabolic state caused by fever and replaces fluid lost with diaphoresis or insensible loss via lungs; vascular volume important for transfer of heat to skin surface
Provide comfortable room temperature; extra covers if needed	Promotes comfort and prevents chilling which increases heat production by muscles when shivering occurs

Information, Instruction, Demonstration

Interventions	Rationales
Report temperature elevation of over 100°F	Prevents difficulty in reducing temperature and possible damage to organs
Oral temperature measurement	Permits self-care and control over care

Discharge or Maintenance Evaluation

- Antipyretic effective in reducing and maintaining baseline temperature
- Temperature at baseline levels within 48 hours
- Absence of chilling, skin pink in color and moist to touch
- I&O ratio in balance

Knowledge deficit

Related to: Lack of information (avoidance of complications or recurrence of disease)
Defining characteristics: Verbalization of the problem, statement of misconception, request for information

Outcome Criteria

Appropriate knowledge of preventative measures and procedures that may decrease severity, the spread of inflammation, infection or reoccurrence of disease.

Interventions	Rationales
Assess knowledge of influenza, methods to prevent acquiring or transmitting disease	Prevents repetition of information; promotes compliance of necessary self-care procedures
Careful handwashing procedure	Removes transient microortanisms
Wear mask, avoid exposure to people with URI	Prevents inhalation of airborne virus
Limit visitors during most acute phase	Prevents additional exposure to microorganisms
Allow for longer bedrest and convalescence if heart or lung disease present	Additional risk for pneumonia or other complication
Suggest influenza immunization in fall before flu season; inform of side effects	Elderly in high risk group are recommended to receive flu vaccine

Discharge or Maintenance Evaluation

- Discusses concerns about past episodes with disease and fears about recurrence and possible complication
- Verbalizes interest and readiness to learn
- Asks questions, requests information
- Follows through on instructions in precautionary measures
- Receives influenza immunization yearly
- Absence of flu symptoms
- Absence of bloody or purulent sputum, changes in breathing from baseline

Pneumonia

An acute infection of the lung tissue that includes the bronchioles and alveoli. It is considered an important cause of death in the elderly, especially those with debilitating diseases. Of the three types of pneumonia, bronchopneumonia is considered to be the most common in the elderly because of a decline in immunity and a presence of other diseases that predispose them to this condition.

MEDICAL CARE

Anti-infectives: penicillins: ampicillin (Amcil), amoxicillin (Amoxil), nafcillin (Nafcil) PO to prevent bacterial cell wall synthesis; **cephalosporins:** cephalexin (Keflex), cefuroxime axetil (Ceftin) PO to destroy organisms by binding to proteins on cell wall inhibiting cell wall synthesis; **aminoglycosides:** gentamicin (Garamycin), tobramycin (Nebcin) PO by inhibiting protein biosynthesis; **other:** erythromycin (Eryc) PO to prevent cell wall synthesis

Expectorants: guaifenesin (Robitussin) PO to irritate gastric mucosa to stimulate gastric reflex and production of respiratory secretions

Antitussives: dextromethorphan (Romilar) PO to act on cough center in medulla to suppress cough

Analgesics, Antipyretics: acetaminophen (Tylenol) aspirin (Bayer) PO to reduce temperature by action on hypothalamus; to control, treat pain by action on CNS pathways

Flu, Pneumovax vaccine: Injections to provide immunity to influenza and pneumonia in those at risk

Chest x-ray: Reveals areas affected by consolidation

Sputum culture: To identify infectious agent and anti-infective sensitivity

CBC: Increases in WBC resulting from infection

NURSING CARE PLANS

Essential nursing diagnoses and plans associated with this condition:

Ineffective airway clearance (44)

Related to: Tracheobronchial infection, obstruction
Defining characteristics: Changes in rate, depth of respirations, ineffective cough, stasis of secretions, crackles, cyanosis

Ineffective breathing pattern (45)

Related to: Pain (pleuritic)
Defining characteristics: Respiratory depth changes

Related to: Inflammatory process (microbial invasion)
Defining characteristics: Tachypnea, cough, crackles

Altered nutrition: less than body requirements (118)

Related to: Inability to ingest foods caused by biological factors
Defining characteristics: Anorexia, lack of interest in food, weakness, weight loss

Impaired physical mobility (196)

Related to: Intolerance to activity
Defining characteristics: Weakness, fatigue, decreased strength and endurance, imposed bedrest, pain

Pneumonia

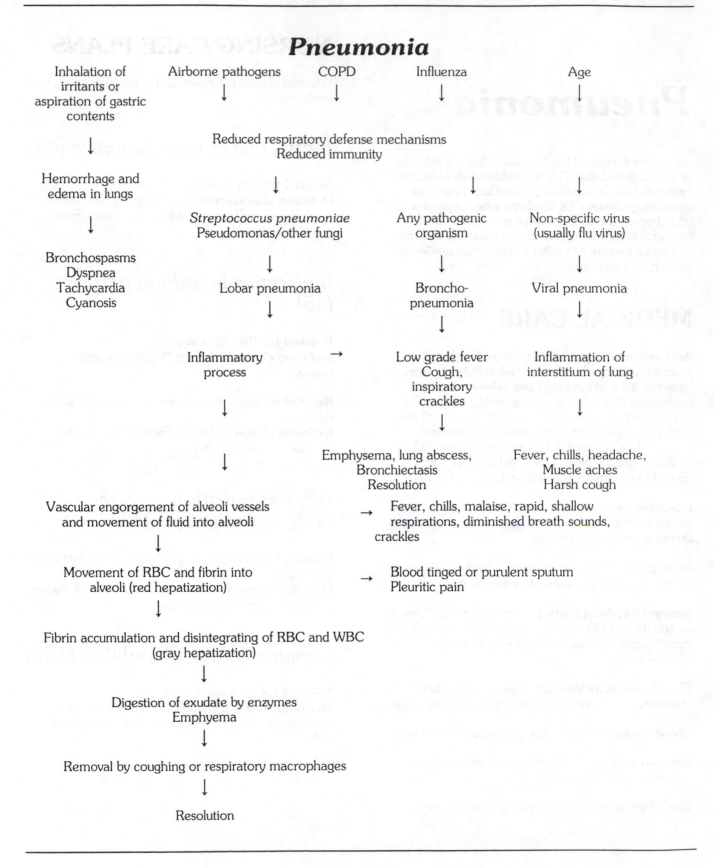

Inhalation of irritants or aspiration of gastric contents

↓

Hemorrhage and edema in lungs

↓

Bronchospasms
Dyspnea
Tachycardia
Cyanosis

Airborne pathogens   COPD   Influenza   Age

↓   ↓   ↓   ↓

Reduced respiratory defense mechanisms
Reduced immunity

↓

Streptococcus pneumoniae   Any pathogenic   Non-specific virus
Pseudomonas/other fungi   organism   (usually flu virus)

↓   ↓   ↓

Lobar pneumonia   Broncho-   Viral pneumonia
                                 pneumonia

↓   ↓   ↓

Inflammatory   →   Low grade fever   Inflammation of
process   Cough,   interstitium of lung
                               inspiratory
                                crackles

↓   ↓   ↓

                           Emphysema, lung abscess,   Fever, chills, headache,
                               Bronchiectasis   Muscle aches
                                Resolution   Harsh cough

Vascular engorgement of alveoli vessels   →   Fever, chills, malaise, rapid, shallow
and movement of fluid into alveoli   respirations, diminished breath sounds,
                                                crackles

↓

Movement of RBC and fibrin into   →   Blood tinged or purulent sputum
alveoli (red hepatization)   Pleuritic pain

↓

Fibrin accumulation and disintegrating of RBC and WBC
(gray hepatization)

↓

Digestion of exudate by enzymes
Emphyema

↓

Removal by coughing or respiratory macrophages

↓

Resolution

SPECIFIC DIAGNOSES AND CARE PLANS

Pain

Related to: Biological injuring agent (infectious process)
Defining characteristics: Communication of pain descriptors

Outcome Criteria

Relief or absence of pleuritic pain.

Interventions	Rationales
Assess presence of pleuritic pain, harsh coughing	Results from inflammation of interstitium or movement of fluid, RBC and fibrin into alveoli of lung
Administer analgesic and antitussive	Relieves pain and coughing
Splint chest during coughing with pillow	Stabilizes chest and prevents pain
Change position q2h using hands or pillow to splint chest	Relieves painful movements while relieving pressure on skin

Discharge or Maintenance Evaluation

- Analgesic or non-analgesic methods to reduce pain and promote comfort
- Verbalizes that pain is eliminated during coughing, movement or deep breathing

Hyperthermia

Related to: Illness (lung inflammation/infection)

Defining characteristics: Low grade or high elevation in body temperature above normal range

Outcome Criteria

Temperature reduced to baseline level.

Interventions	Rationales
Assess temperature elevations above 96.8°F (37°C), chills malaise, muscle aches	Systemic response to inflammation as body increases blood flow and metabolism to assist healing
Administer antipyretic	Prevents extreme elevations to protect vulnerable organs such as the brain
Administer anti-infectives specific to identified organism	Destroys organisms by inhibiting cell wall synthesis
Sponge with cool cloth with care to avoid chilling	Increases heat loss by evaporation
Comfortable environmental temperature; provide extra covers	Promotes comfort and prevents chilling
Increase fluid intake up to 2-3 L/day (10-12 glasses), offer ice chips, popsicles, juices of choice	Replaces fluid loss from diaphoresis and prevents dehydration
Change damp linens or clothing as needed if diaphoretic	Promotes comfort and prevents further chilling

Information, Instruction, Demonstration

Interventions	Rationales
Taking oral temperature measurement	Permits independence in monitoring temperature

Discharge or Maintenance Evaluation

- Antipyretic and/or non-pharmaceutical measures effective in reducing and maintaining baseline temperature
- I&O ratio in balance
- Temperature at baseline levels within 48-72 hours with anti-infective therapy

Risk for injury

Related to: External biological factor of micro-organism transmission, internal developmental factor of aging process

Defining characteristics: Over 65 years of age, presence of chronic respiratory disease, exposure to causative organisms, complication of pneumonia

Outcome Criteria

Prevention of relapse, reinfection or spread of infectious process.

Interventions	Rationales
Assess presence of a chronic condition, history of past episodes of pneumonia or acute respiratory conditions	Elderly with chronic illnesses more susceptible to respiratory infections with increased morbidity
Assess knowledge of precautionary measures to prevent infection	Prevents acquiring or transmitting the disease; provides for teaching strategies
Carry out proper handwashing before giving care, wear mask if appropriate	Prevents cross-contamination and exposure of client to infectious agents
Regulate visitors who have URI	Prevents superimposed infections
Provide private room, protective isolation if appropriate	Prevents transmission of organisms to client and optimal environment for rest/sleep

Information, Instruction, Demonstration

Interventions	Rationales
Handwashing technique	Prevents transmission of organisms by hands
Use of covered container for sputum and proper disposal of tissues	Prevents spread via contaminated articles
Suggest Pneumovax vaccination; inform of potential for recurrence	Provides lifelong immunization against bacterial pneumonia

Discharge or Maintenance Evaluation

- Carries out precautionary measures to prevent spread of infection or recurrence
- Avoids those with URI infections especially during winter months
- Acquires immunization for pneumonia
- Resolution of disease without complications (empyema)

Neurological System

Neurological System

Alteration in the central nervous system affects the integrative abilities associated with aging. The system responds to changes in the circulatory system (atherosclerosis) because of its need for oxygen. Changes in the supply of oxygen to the brain causes changes in mentation, sensory perception, movement and the ability to cope with multiple environmental stimuli. The changes and their manifestations vary with individuals. One can, however, expect a decline in sensory-motor flexibility while intellectual function, verbal comprehension remain the same or increase. The rate and persistance of the changes in structure and function of the CNS brought about by the aging process and changes that occur in the other systems determine the degree of deficit or deprivation in an individual client.

GENERAL NEUROLOGICAL CHANGES ASSOCIATED WITH THE AGING PROCESS

Brain structure

- Weight loss of brain with aging causing reduction in number of neurons with a greater loss in some areas of cortex and cerebellum
- Atrophy of convolutions with widening sulci and gyri mostly in frontal lobe
- Dilitation of the ventricles as aging progresses
- Increased intracellular accumulation of lipofuscin pigment causing nuclei in cells to assume an abnormal position
- Development of senile plaques or anatomic lesions with aging

Metabolic and physiologic function

- Decreased oxygen consumption causing decreased intracellular energy, glucose utilization, blood flow
- Metabolic changes within synaptic complexes causing neurotransmitter effects related to brain function of sleep, temperature control, mood resulting in sleep disturbance, cold intolerance and depression
- Reduced levels of norepinephrine, increased levels of serotonin and monoamine oxidase causing changes in neurotransmitter function and depression; decreased dopamine level causing Parkinson's disease
- General changes related to cerebral circulation causing changes in mental acuity (association, retrieval, recall, memory, cognitive ability), in movement (motor strength, agility, dexterity), in sensory interpretation (sight, hearing, taste, smell, touch), in capacity to cope with multiple events (depression, affect, communication)
- Decreased number of neurons causing a decrease in transmission strength from brain to body parts and resulting in altered threshold for arousal of organ or system
- Increased recovery time of autonomic nervous system causing longer time to return to baseline organ function after stimulation resulting in anxiety and tension from overstimulation
- Decrease in deep tendon reflex intensity in arms, absence of ankle reflexes, absent plantar reflex in presence of foot problems
- Decreases in dendrites in nerve, synapses, lesions on axons causing decrease in peripheral nerve conduction and slow reaction time
- Extrapyramidal changes causing changes in affect, reduced movement and blinking

Electroencephalographic changes

- Readings reveal one cycle lower than in other adult stages

Sensory structure and function

- Pupils decrease in size and are less responsive to intensity in light alterations causing difficulty in seeing in dark, at night or a slower adaptation to the dark
- The irises acquire more density of pigmentation
- Decrease in sensitivity of cones in retina to color causing difficulty in discriminating changes in color and blending of colors at opposite ends of the color spectrum (red and green becomes black)
- A pattern of dark spots or clouds in red reflex seen with ophthalmological examination
- Constriction response slightly delayed
- Loss of fat cushion around eye causing globe to sink deeper into socket; lids become thinner and wrinkled
- Decreased secretion by lacrimal glands causing the conjunctiva to become dry and lack luster; tiny, red vessels may be visible
- Sclera becomes yellower and may have pigmented deposits
- Cornea may develop white-yellow deposits at periphery (arcus senilis), becomes less translucent and more spherical
- The anterior chamber becomes shallower causing potential for glaucoma
- Yellowish plaques may appear near inner canthus (xanthelasma)
- Lenses lose elasticity and become opaque causing potential for cataract formation, reduced focus and accommodation, loss of peripheral vision, decreased tolerance to glare, decreased ability to differentiate visual detail and colors, decreased night vision. Yellowing of the lens makes vision for blues and greens more difficult.
- Sclerosis or atrophy of tympanic membrane, increased rigidity of bones of middle ear causing difficulty hearing high frequency sounds (tone discrimination), hearing if noise is present,

sound distortion, phonetic regression. Cerumen contains greater amounts of keratin which makes it harder and easily impacted.
- Deterioration of sense of smell, touch and reduction in number of taste buds causing a gradual loss which decreases pain, pressure, hot/cold perception, anorexia and disinterest in food

Sleep changes

- Remains in stages I and II for longer period of time and may require longer time to fall asleep
- Stage III remains the same, stage IV time is greatly reduced or skipped altogether with aging causing more frequent wakenings at night and a decreased intensity of sleep making it easier to be awakened and an impression of not getting enough sleep
- REM sleep time is comparable to other stages of adulthood but aging results in less dreaming and a reduction in REM causes irritability, lethargy, depression
- Reduction in stage IV causing feeling of fatigue, tiredness, anxiety and tension
- Insomnia, sleep apnea and napping increase with age causing sleep pattern disturbances and deprivation

ESSENTIAL DIAGNOSES AND CARE PLANS

Altered thought processes

Related to: Physiological changes
Defining characteristics: Cognitive dissonance, decreased ability to grasp ideas, impaired ability to make decisions, impaired ability to problem solve, impaired ability to reason, impaired ability to conceptualize, impaired ability to calculate, altered attention span-distractibility, inability to follow commands, disorientation to time, place, person, circumstances and events

Related to: Psychological conflicts
Defining characteristics: Egocentricity, hyper/hypovigilance, obsessions, delusions, hallucinations, inappropriate social behavior

Related to: Loss of memory
Defining characteristics: Memory deficit or problems, changes in remote, recent, immediate memory, ideas of reference

Related to: Sleep deprivation
Defining characteristics: Altered sleep pattern, lethargy, disorientation, confusion, cognitive dissonance

Outcome Criteria

Maintenance of mental and psychological function and reversal of behaviors when possible.

Interventions	Rationales
Assess cognitive functioning, memory changes, thinking pattern, disorientation, sleep and communication difficulty	Mental process influenced by metabolic and physiologic changes associated with aging
Assess state of confusion, ability to make judgments, presence of delusions, illusions, hallucination, restlessness, anxiety, depression, increased introversion, quarreling	Confusion level may range from slight disorientation to uncooperation to agitation and develops over short period of time or slowly over periods of months
Assess ability to cope with events, making negative remarks, interest, motivation, assertiveness or aggressiveness, changes in memory pattern	Elderly have a decrease in memory for more recent events and a more active memory for past events and reminiscence about the pleasant ones, may become more assertive to compensate for feelings of insecurity, develop more narrowed interests and have difficulty accepting changes in lifestyle

Interventions	Rationales
Assess for sensory deprivation, use of CNS drugs, presence of poor nutrition, dehydration, metabolic/neurologic/cardiac/pulmonary disorders or infection	May cause confusion and mental changes
Provide orientation during each interaction in slow and calm manner	Provides reality and prevents frustration with a memory loss and diminished ability to decipher messages
Provide clocks, calendars, address by name	Fills memory gaps
Maintain regular daily schedule	Predictable behavior is less threatening and does not tax limited ability in functioning in ADL
Allow to sit in chair near window; offer TV, newspaper, books as appropriate	Assists to differentiate between day and night and promote reality of environment
Label drawers, write reminder note, use pictures or color code for access to articles	Aids memory by utilizing reminders of what to do and location of articles, rooms
Respect personal space and provide privacy when needed	Less threatening and allows for some control
Allow hoarding, wandering in a controlled environment	Increases security and permits behaviors that are difficult to prevent in a safe, supervised environment; decreases hostility and agitation
Focus on positive behavior, give positive feedback, use familiar events to praise competence	Capitalizes on progress and promotes confidence

Interventions	Rationales
Introduce new ideas, any staff changes and activities slowly with time for gradual adaptation	Narrowing interests cause difficulty in accepting new ideas or changes
Provide opportunity for reminiscence while maintaining reality	Allows for memory of past pleasant events
Limit sensory input and decisions to be made unless able to maintain own role, involvement in activities and independent decision making	Decreases frustration and distractions from environment; self-assertive attitude may be channeled and promote security
Convey warmth and concern during care and communications	Feelings of loneliness, isolation and depression are common
Provide social involvement with others; encourage but avoid forcing interactions; consider day care center if appropriate	Prevents isolation, loss of reality
Repeat information when needed; provide distractions or change subject if repetitive speech occurs or becomes argumentative or overly sensitive	Changes train of thought and promotes understanding without feeding into undesirable behavior

Discharge or Maintenance Evaluation

- Mental functional abilities at optimum level with modifications and alterations in environment to compensate for deficits
- Thought processes improved or maintained at baseline level
- Awareness of environment and orientation preserved and reality maintained at optimum level
- Psychological conflicts controlled and behavior identified and improved

- Achievement of highest level of mental and psychological function

Sensory/perceptual alterations: visual, auditory, kinesthetic, gustatory, tactile, olfactory

Related to: Altered sensory reception, transmission and/or integration of neurological disease or deficit, altered status of sense organs, inability to communicate, understand, speak or respond, sleep deprivation
Defining characteristics: Disorientation in time, place, person, reported or measured change in sensory acuity, altered abstraction, conceptualization, change in problem solving abilities, apathy, complaints of fatigue, altered communication patterns, lack of, or poor concentration, noncompliance, disordered thought sequencing, visual and auditory distortions, motor incoordination, posture alterations

Related to: Chemical alteration of hypoxia, CNS stimulants or depressants, mind altering drugs
Defining characteristics: Change in behavior pattern, change in usual response to stimuli, apathy, restlessness, rapid mood swings, exaggerated emotional responses, bizarre thinking, inappropriate responses

Related to: Environmental factor of socially restricted institutionalization, aging, chronic illness
Defining characteristics: Disorientation, change in behavior pattern, anxiety, apathy, exaggerated emotional responses, anger, irritability, depression, rapid mood swings

Outcome Criteria

Preservation of sensory/perceptual function and controlled effects of deficits.

Interventions	Rationales	Interventions	Rationales
Assess for confusion state, disorientation, difficulty and slowing of mental ability, changes in behavior and emotional responses	Cognitive dysfunction behavior change may result from sensory deficits/deprivation caused by physiological, psychological and environmental factors	Administer mydriatics, miotics as eye drops	Mydriatics act to improve vision with cataracts; miotics facilitate flow of aqueous humor through canal of Schlemm
Assess visual acuity, visual difficulties and loss and effects from these changes (withdrawal, isolation), presence of cataract, glaucoma, macular degeneration and status of remaining vision	Presbyopia common in elderly, other visual changes caused by physiological changes require correction by surgery, eye glasses; visual deficits create mobility and socialization changes	Administer softening agent to ear and irrigate with bulb syringe or low pulsating water pick	Softens cerumen buildup and emulsifies it for easier removal to facilitate hearing
		Promote use of assistive devices, hearing aid or corrective glasses, contact lenses	Provides for correction of deficit
Assess auditory acuity, cerumen in ears, responses to noises and effect on hearing, ability to communicate, amount of loss and effect, difficulty in locating and identifying sounds	Presbycusis common in elderly, conductive loss results in a false interpretation of the world and creates poor communication, isolation, depression, impaired thought processes as interactions are not heard	Provide reading materials with large print, recorded material, telephone with large numbers, posters with contrasting colors	Provides for visual aids that allow for more control and independence
		Provide magnifying glass, reading stand with magnifier attached, brighter lighting	Promotes visual acuity
Assess olfactory/gustatory loss, changes in appetite and eating, amount of loss and effect on nutritional status	Deterioration results from physiological changes of aging and creates loss of interest and pleasure of eating	Suggest sunglasses or visor; change intensity of light evenly whether increasing or decreasing	Reduces glare that is common complaint in elderly
Assess tactile changes, tingling or numbness in extremities, loss of sensations is decreased cold, pain, pressure	Tactile perception reduced in aged and discriminating different sensations is decreased and creates risk of injury	Arrange articles in familiar fashion and maintain same location; follow through with food on table, personal hygiene articles, clothing, furniture	Provides alteration in environment that facilitates independence with limited vision; promotes safety
Assess kinesthetic perception, expression or behavior indicating awareness, extent and direction of movement	Cognitive deficits or aging neurologic changes may prevent awareness, control of muscles, muscle movements and creates risk of falls	Suggest to use colors that are bright and contrasting; avoid blues and greens	Minimizes problem of distinguishing items from one another as colors tend to blend
		Provide for adequate lighting at night; avoid abrupt movement from too much light to too little light	Prevents confusion and accidents as ability to adjust to differences in lighting is decreased

Interventions	Rationales
Provide telephone amplifier on receiver and bell tone, flashing light on phone, loud speakers for TV, radio, tape and CD players	Promotes auditory perception and acuity
Determine type of hearing loss, if head turned to hear, asks for repeat of conversations frequently, inability to follow verbal conversation	The elderly with conductive loss experiences loss of hearing all frequencies and will hear any loudly spoken words; sensorineural loss experiences loss of hearing even when speech is loud enough to be heard
Eliminate background noise	Interferes with hearing
Face the client, use eye contact and speak loudly enough to be heard, speak slowly and clearly with proper pitch, use short sentences and gestures, maintain position even with client to allow view of lips, use touch to hold attention	Enhances communication if hearing impaired and promotes feelings of warmth and caring
Allow time for answers, rephrase message using different words if confused, puzzled or gives inappropriate response	May need time to sort out and identify sounds or may not understand certain frequency sounds
Use smaller groups, room with carpet, drapes	Promotes communication by reducing echoes
Use hand-held device if appropriate	Hearing horns and speaking tubes enhance communication
Offer sweet and salt substitutes	Satisfies desire for these tastes as taste buds decrease with aging without compromising special dietary regimens

Interventions	Rationales
Allow for interaction during mealtime	Promotes interest in eating
Provide alarm and flashing light type smoke detector, safety alarms for stoves, heating units	Reduces risk of injury if olfactory perception is reduced
Prevent any exposure to extreme temperatures, pressure to skin	Reduces risk of burns or injury if tactile perception impaired
Provide assistance when ambulating or performing ADL as appropriate	Reduces risk of falls or injury if visual acuity reduced or if kinesthetic perception impaired
Encourage participation in physical/social interactions	Prevents isolation and sensory deficit

Information, Instruction, Demonstration

Interventions	Rationales
Application of eye and/or ear medication; stress importance of drug therapy compliance	Preserves visual acuity and prevents visual loss; promotes auditory acuity
Cleansing of glasses with mild soap and warm water and drying with lint free cloth	Promotes vision through clean glasses
Applying, removing hearing device weekly and cleaning ear and device and troubleshoot according to manufacturer's instruction pamphlet	Prevents cerumen accumulation and enhances hearing
Suggest yearly vision and hearing testing	Provides for adjustments in corrective devices

Interventions	Rationales
Environmental modifications to enhance vision, hearing, taste, smell, touch as appropriate	Safety precautions prevent injury in presence of sensory impairment
Consider pet therapy	Provides stimulation and touch enhancement; facilitates interaction
Inform that time is needed to adapt to assistive aids	Established patterns take time to change
Inform of groups to assist blind, deaf	Assists with information, programs, books, tapes, and other resources for the deaf and blind
Reinforce information about aging changes that affect sensory and cognitive perception	Promotes understanding of deficit and motivates to implement measures that improve function

Discharge or Maintenance Evaluation

- Identifies sounds and objects correctly
- Uses assistive aids to maximize deficits; statements of ability to hear/see with use of devices
- Administers eye and ear medications correctly and complies with medication regimen
- Adjustments made in environment with prevention of accidents/confusion
- Adjustments made to enhance vision, hearing, taste, smell perception
- Intraocular pressure increases prevented
- Early recognition of changes or increased impairment of sensory perception and periodic participation in tests
- Cleanses and cares for assistive devices properly

Impaired verbal communication

Related to: Decrease in circulation to brain
Defining characteristics: Dyspnea, disorientation, inability to speak

Related to: Age related factors
Defining characteristics: Sensory deficits, does not or cannot speak, stuttering, slurring, impaired articulation, difficulty with phonation, inability to find, name words, inability to identify objects

Related to: Psychological barriers, psychosis, lack of stimuli
Defining characteristics: Loose association of ideas, flight of ideas, incessant verbalization, disorientation, confusion, impaired social interaction

Outcome Criteria

Effective speech and understanding or alternative method to communicate needs verbally or nonverbally.

Interventions	Rationales
Assess speech ability, language deficit, cognitive or sensory impairment, presence of aphasia, dysarthia, hypoxia, presence of psychosis, neurological disorder affecting speech	Identifies strengths and unusual speech patterns
Assess effect of communication deficit (isolation or disengagement, agitation, frustration, depression)	Speech and language deficit are result of changes in the dominant hemisphere of the brain (most commonly the left) and poses one of the most difficult problems for the elderly as they are not able to make their needs known which leads to psychosocial behavior changes

Interventions	Rationales
Assess nonverbal communication (grimaces, smiles, pointing, frowning, crying) and encourage use until speech improves or returns	Indicates feelings or needs when speech impaired
Anticipate and validate needs as appropriate	Prevents frustration and anxiety
Provide calm, unhurried attitude and environment; avoid competing noises or stimuli	Allows for uninterrupted attention without distractions
When speaking, face client, speak slowly and distinctly in moderate or low-pitched tone	Clarity, brevity and time for response promotes chance for successful speech
Ask simple, direct questions that require short yes or no answers; repeat or reword misunderstood statements	Promotes self-confidence
Listen actively to interpret message and confirm with client	Facilitates communication
Use gestures, facial expressions, pantomine, pictures, lists or demonstrate what is to be done	Provides information and method to send and receive messages
Encourage speech effort; avoid criticism and accept behavior resulting from frustration	Promotes but doesn't force or make judgements about speech attempts
Encourage to take time when attempting speech, to speak loudly, slowly and distinctly as if listener is deaf and in short phrases, use of nonverbal gestures with speech attempts	Reaction time is reduced and voice volume may decline; understanding enhanced when stress reduced and word and sentence usage are concise

Interventions	Rationales
Provide pencil and paper, magic slate, typewriter to write messages	Alternate methods of communication if fine motor function present
Encourage practice of facial muscle exercise by smiling, frowning, extending tongue out and moving it up, down, sideways	Promotes facial expressions used for communication by improving muscle integrity and coordination
Encourage to breathe before speaking, pausing between words and use tongue, lips and jaw to speak	Promotes coordinated speech and breathing
Encourage to control length and rate of phrases, overarticulate words and separate syllables and emphasize consonants	Promotes speech in presence of dysarthria

Information, Instruction, Demonstration

Interventions	Rationales
Advise to use glasses, hearing aid, dentures as appropriate	Enhances communication in presence of sensory or other deficit
Refer to speech pathologist	Promotes facilitation of remaining speech ability or provides alternatives
Practice exercises daily	Strengthens facial muscles
Practice verbal communication such as reading menu aloud	Enhances speech skills

Discharge or Maintenance Evaluation

- Uses aids or techniques to facilitate communication
- Speaks in understandable way when possible
- Able to understand communications
- Maximizes ability to communicate needs
- Minimal anxiety and frustration with speech attempts
- Progressive return of speech to baseline determinations when appropriate

Sleep pattern disturbance

Related to: Internal factor of illness (cardiac, pulmonary, renal, thyroid)
Defining characteristics: Interrupted sleep, difficulty falling asleep, awakening early, fatigue, lethargy, irritability, disorientation, complaints of not feeling rested

Related to: Psychological stress (depression, confusion, boredom)
Defining characteristics: Insomnia, sleeplessness, naps during day, fatigue, lethargy, disorientation, expressionless face

Related to: External factor of environmental changes (stimuli, obstructive sleep apnea)
Defining characteristics: Interrupted sleep, exhaustion, snoring, long periods of silence, cessation of breathing, sleepiness during day, yawning, lethargy, morning headache, loss of libido

Outcome Criteria

Maintenance of restorative, restful sleep.

Interventions	Rationales
Assess sleep pattern and changes, naps and frequency, amount of activity or sedentary status, awakenings and when they occur and frequency, feelings of fatigue, apathy, lethargy, impotence	Provides data for resolving sleep deprivation in relation to aging changes
Assess presence of pain, dyspnea, nocturia, leg cramps	Causes of frequent awakenings and interruptions in sleep
Assess presence of depression, boredom, confusion, dementia, obesity, chronic anxiety	Common causes of insomnia and sleep pattern disturbance
Assess use of sedatives, alcohol, caffeine, medication regimen	Alters REM sleep which may cause irritability, lethargy; drug action, absorption and excretion may be delayed in elderly and adverse effects and toxicity at higher risk
Assess environment for lighting, noises, odors, temperature, ventilation	External stimuli interferes with going to sleep and increases wakenings as sleep in the elderly is of less intensity
Provide ritualistic procedures of warm drink, extra covers, clean linens, warm bath before bedtime	Prevents break in established pattern and promotes comfort and relaxation before sleep
Provide calm, quiet, peaceful environment	Promotes falling asleep
Allow naps during day according to need recognizing that they may interfere with sleep and cause insomnia	Some elderly prefer to sleep throughout 24 hours with short naps providing adequate rest

Interventions	Rationales
Provide backrub, relaxation techniques, imagery, music, massage at bedtime	Promotes relaxation before sleep and reduces anxiety and tension
Provide sleep apnea apparatus and position for sleep	Allows for completion of all stages of sleep resulting in restorative sleep

Information, Instruction, Demonstration

Interventions	Rationales
Refrain from use of sedatives, alcohol, CNS depressants	Depresses REM sleep and may take 5-8 weeks for normal sleep pattern to return
Inform of aging changes and their relation to sleep changes	Assists in acceptance of changes and need for revision of sleep pattern
Avoid stimulation before sleep such as caffeine drinks, excessive activity, stressful events or interactions	Prevents falling asleep because of overstimulation
Instruct in weight reduction diet if appropriate	Obesity predisposes to sleep apnea

Discharge or Maintenance Evaluation

- Develops sleep pattern including naps that results in rested feeling and absence of fatigue, lethargy, sleepiness
- Modifications of environment, reduced use of drugs and stimulation, use of apnea apparatus to promote restorative sleep
- Statements that physical and mental changes and symptoms reduced as adequate sleep attained

Alzheimer's Disease/ Dimentia Disorders

The progressive, reversible or irreversible deterioration of mental functioning resulting from organic pathology is know as dementia. It can be permanent or temporary depending on the underlying abnormal condition or disease that can be associated with it. The most common forms of dementia are Alzheimer's disease in which the cause is unknown, and multi-infarct which results from vascular disorders. Alzheimer's disease, Parkinson's disease, Huntington's disease, and Pick's disease are examples of irreversible dementias. Depression, multiple sclerosis, brain infections and other disorders, abnormalities resulting from hypertension (stroke) or diabetes (hypo or hyperglycemia), anemia, thyroid disorders, malnutrition, and medication-related are examples of reversible dementias.

Alzheimer's disease is characterized by a progressive deterioration of mental, motor, and emotional capabilities. This type of dementia uses the title of dementia of the Alzheimer type (DAT) to define it since it is a type of dementia that is the same regardless of age as opposed to multi-infarct or reversible dementias. Stages identify the disease progression beginning with memory impairment, speech and motor difficulties, to disorientation to time and place, impaired judgement, memory loss, forgetfulness and inappropriate affect (lasts 2-4 years), followed by loss of independence, complete disorientation, wandering, hoarding, communication difficulties, complete memory loss (lasts up to 7 years), and the final stage with blank expression, irritability, seizures, emaciation, and absolute depend-

ence (last year) until death. The total duration of the disease is estimated to be 14 years.

Multi-infarct dementia progresses as new lesions appear in the brain and is characterized by emotional lability, dysarthria, weakness, hyperreflexia, dysphagia, changes in cognitive function (memory, thinking, judgement), confusion, delirium, and instability of emotional responses.

Dementias resulting from reversible causes are characterized by cognitive impairment, memory loss, depression, hypochondriasis, confusion, lethargy, loss of control of behavior.

MEDICAL CARE

Sedative/Hypnotic (Barbituate): amobarbital (Amytal sodium) PO to promote sleep when sleep cycles have been disrupted in dementia conditions

Cholinesterase inhibitor: tacrine or THA (Cognex) PO to improve cognitive function in Alzheimer's disease

Antipsychotic: thiothixene (Navane), trifluoperazine (Stelazine) PO for management of agitation, aggressive behavior in dementia conditions

CT scan: Reveals brain atrophy and enlargement of the ventricles later in the disease

NURSING CARE PLANS

Essential nursing diagnoses and plans associated with this condition:

Altered thought processes (70)

Related to: Physiological changes of cognitive ability, impaired memory, disorientation

Alzheimer's Disease

← Aging, genetic factors →

↓ ↓ ↓ ↓

| Neurofibrillary tangles and filaments wrapped around each other and neurons in cerebral cortex | Loss of neurons
Cerebral atrophy
Widening sulci
Senile plaques
Reduced water matter
Ventricular dilation
Granulovascular bodies | Inadequate blood flow to brain | Decreased acetylcholinesterase and choline acetyltransferase |

↓ ↓ ↓ ↓

→ Memory impairment ←
Decreased intellectual functioning
Forgetfulness
Confusion

↓

Cognitive impairment
Deterioration in personal habits/social behavior
Aphasia, apraxia, agnosia
Hyperexcitability
Gait disturbance

↓

Total dependence

↓

Death

Defining characteristics: Decreased ability to reason, conceptualize, memory loss, deterioration in personal care and appearance, dysarthia, dysphagia, convulsions

Related to: Psychological conflicts from dementia
Defining characteristics: Inappropriate social behavior, paranoia, combativeness, uncooperation, wandering, disturbance in memory, judgement, abstract thought, explosive behavior, illusions, delusions, hallucinations, deterioration in intellectual capability, loss of sexual drive and interest, reduced control of sexual behavior (masturbation and exposure in public, inappropriate advances)

Impaired verbal communication (75)

Related to: Psychological barriers, psychosis from dementia
Defining characteristics: Confusion, anxiety, restlessness, disorientation to person, place, event, and time, incessant verbalization with repetitive speech, agitation, flight of ideas

Sleep pattern disturbance (77)

Related to: Psychological stress from depression, confusion, effect of medications
Defining characteristics: Insomnia, disorientation, restlessness, frequent awakenings, anxiety, excessive daytime naps, impaired communication

Functional incontinence (154)

Related to: Sensory, cognitive deficits causing inability to respond to urge
Defining characteristics: Urinary/fecal incontinence, changes in voiding (dysuria, frequency), inadequate fluid intake, inability to recognize or reach toilet

Altered nutrition: less than body requirements (118)

Related to: Inability to ingest food because of biological factors of dysphagia
Defining characteristics: Difficulty swallowing, weight loss, decreased cough and gag reflex, confusion, inability to feed self, food left in mouth

SPECIFIC DIAGNOSES AND CARE PLANS

Self-care deficit: bathing, hygiene, dressing, grooming

Related to: Perceptual or cognitive impairment (memory loss, confusion)
Defining characteristics: Inability to wash body or body parts, inability to put on or take off necessary clothing, fasten clothing, inability to maintain appearance at satisfactory level

Related to: Neuromuscular impairment (gait disturbance)
Defining characteristics: Inability to obtain clothing, inability to get to water source

Outcome Criteria

Appropriately bathed, groomed and dressed independently or with assistance.

Interventions	Rationales
Assess appearance, body odors, ability to recognize and use articles for washing and grooming, specific self-care deficits	Provides specific care needs and amount of help needed; middle stages of disease is best time to encourage independence and decision-making

Interventions	Rationales
Arrange to provide care similar to previous patterns using familiar equipment and maintain consistency in daily activities of bathing, grooming and hygiene	Promotes familiarity and prevents further confusion and agitation
Lay out articles and clothing in order of use	Promotes independence and ease in self-care without causing agitation or frustration
Provide clothing with velcro closings, zippers, elastic waist, large neck to slip over head or open in front	Promotes ease in dressing
Provide hand bars, mat in tub and check water temperature	Safety devices to prevent falls and burns
Allow time to perform each task, avoid rushing or adhering to schedule; remind of activity when needed	Promotes self-care for as long as possible
Assist with as much of activity as needed, show patience in allowing for free movement and avoid trying to reason with client	Promotes independence andself esteem when allowed control over situations

Information, Instruction, Demonstration

Interventions	Rationales
Instruct in activity with a step-by-step method without rushing	Promotes self-esteem and feeling of accomplishment

Interventions	Rationales
Demonstrate use of each article of care; toothbrush, tooth paste, soap, wash cloth, towel, deodorant, comb or hairbrush	Promotes self-care and enhances appearance

Discharge or Maintenance Evaluation

- Acceptable appearance
- Participation in ADL within neurological limitations
- Accepts assistance in care when needed
- Utilizes assistive aids to perform self-care

Risk for trauma

Related to: Cognitive or emotional difficulties (memory impairment, confusion, decreased intellectual functioning)

Defining characteristics: Gait disturbance, wandering, forgetfulness, impaired judgement, lack of awareness of environmental hazards

Outcome Criteria

Absence of potential for injury.

Interventions	Rationales
Assess mobility and stability, muscle weakness, environmental hazards, cognitive limitations	Causes of trauma from falls or wandering

Interventions	Rationales
Clear pathways, store dangerous objects and substances out of reach, apply alarm system to client to alert that wandering outside of safe limits	Prevents accidental injury to self and others and allows wandering a safe distance rather than restraints or other confinement methods
Place mattress near floor if in danger of falling from bed	Prevents falls from bed, agitation and hostility resulting from restraints
Assist with ambulation when needed, provide rails or other aids for support	Prevents falls
Allow for safe activities when scheduled or desired	Promotes socialization

Information, Instruction, Demonstration

Interventions	Rationales
Refrain from driving car, not capable	Cognitive difficulties during driving may cause injury to client and/or others
Modification of environment to accommodate level of functioning and awareness	Creates safe environment

Discharge or Maintenance Evaluation

- Absence of falls or injury from dangerous objects
- Safety hazards removed
- Wandering within safe environment

Social isolation

Related to: Alterations in mental status (confusion, memory loss)
Defining characteristics: Uncommunicative, withdrawn, absence of support, cognitive impairment, impaired sleep pattern

Related to: Unaccepted social behavior (agitation, combative)
Defining characteristics: Projects hostility in behavior, expresses feelings of rejection, indifference of others, inability to meet expectations of others

Outcome Criteria

Maintain social interaction of client and caregivers with others.

Interventions	Rationales
Assess feelings about behavioral problems, negative feelings about self, ability to communicate, anxiety, depression, feeling of powerlessness	Determines extent of loneliness and isolation and reasons for it
Identify possible support systems and ability to participate in social activities	Community resources available for clients and families dealing with stages of Alzheimer's disease that provide information and assistance
Provide diversional activities as appropriate for functional ability	Provides stimuli and promotes psychosocial functioning
Provide rest and sleep periods; avoid situations that cause frustration or agitation, sensory overload	Permits coping with stimuli and prevents violent reactions

Information, Instruction, Demonstration

Interventions	Rationales
Assist to plan and carry out periods of rest and activities during the day	Provides social activity
Establish consistent bedtime routine; reorient in quiet, calm manner if awakened at night	Promotes sleep and avoids frustration and confusion
Offer list of resources available for assistance	Provides social outlet, financial and psychological counseling

Discharge or Maintenance Evaluation

- Increased participation in social activities
- Statements that there is a reduction in isolation from others
- Utilizes support systems for socialization, counseling
- Statements of satisfactory social relationships

Chronic confusion

Related factors: Alzheimer's disease, multi-infarct dementia, other dementia conditions
Defining characteristics: Organic impairment, altered interpretation/response to stimuli, long-term cognitive impairment, impaired memory and orientation, altered personality

Outcome Criteria

Confusion, cognitive impairment, and other manifestations minimized.

Interventions	Rationales
Assess reversible or irreversible dementia, cause, ability to interpret the environment, intellectual thought, disturbances in orientation, memory, behavior, and socialization	Determines type and extent of dementia to plan and enhance cognitive and emotional functioning
Assess cognitive function with use of Cognitive Rating Scale, Global Deterioration Scale, Alzheimer's Disease Assessment, Clinical Dementia Rating	Rating scales assist to evaluate dementia
Avoid frustrating situation, maintain consistency in schedules, monitor for environmental overstimulation	Prevents agitation, combative reactions or erratic behaviors
Avoid or terminate emotionally charged situations or conversations, avoid anger and expectation of memory or following instructions	Facilitates communication and prevents threat to emotional stability
Collaborate in establishing clues or reminders in daily schedule	Assists to manage memory loss

Information, Instruction, Demonstration

Interventions	Rationales
Provide written and verbal instructions as appropriate	Reminds of important information related to needs
Identify support systems and resources for counseling, social activities	Provides information and assistance to promote functional abilities

Discharge or Maintenance Evaluation

- Maintains stable environment and scheduling of events
- Exhibits minimal or reduction in confusion, memory and cognitive disturbances
- Stimuli tolerated when introduced slowly in a nonthreatening manner
- Consults with professionals for information and support

Ineffective family coping: compromised

Related to: Prolonged disease or disability progression that exhausts supportive capacity of significant people (progressive dementia and dependence of client)

Defining characteristics: Fatigue, chronic anxiety, stress, social isolation, financial insecurity, expression of inadequate understanding of crisis and client's responses to health problem and necessary supportive behaviors

Outcome Criteria

Increased coping ability of client's dementia and care needs.

Interventions	Rationales
Assess knowledge of disease and erratic behaviors, possible violent reactions of client	Knowledge will enhance the family's understanding of the dementia associated with the disease and development of coping skills and strategies

Interventions	Rationales
Assess for level of fatigue, reduced social exposure of family, feelings about role reversal in caring for parent and increasing demands of client	Long-term needs of client may affect physical and psychosocial health of caregiver, economic status and prevent family from achieving own goals in life
Provide for opportunity of family to express concerns and lack of control of situation	Promotes venting of feelings and reduces anxiety
Assist in defining problem and use of techniques to cope and solve problems	Provides support for problem-solving and management of own fatigue and chronic stress
Assist to identify client's reactions and behaviors and reasons for them	May indicate onset of agitation and allow for interventions to prevent or reduce frustration

Information, Instruction, Demonstration

Interventions	Rationales
Demonstrate techniques to assist client with self-care needs of personal hygiene, dressing, eating and toileting	Assists family to provide personal care while conserving their energy
Demonstrate use of aids for walking, protecting the skin, eating, sleeping, remove environmental hazards	Assists family to prevent injury to client
Inform of need to maintain own health, social contacts	Fatigue, isolation, anxiety will affect the physical health and care capabilities of the caregiver

Interventions	Rationales
Suggest community services available for Alzheimer's disease if ready and able to use them; inform of respite care	Offers information and support from those that understand and empathize with families
Suggest social worker referral if appropriate	Provides assistance for economic problems and respite services; long term care facilities need
Inform to contact the Alzheimer's Disease and Related Disorders Association (ADRDA)	Offers support for safety, legal, financial, ethical issues and needs as the disease causes disruption in all aspects of family life

Discharge or Maintenance Evaluation

- Optimal health of family members, caregiver
- Statements of satisfactory contact with support group and/or professionals
- Statements that knowledge about disease and care of client increased and feeling more in control of situation
- Statements that anxiety reduced, coping and problem-solving techniques, relaxation techniques utilized, respite care obtained
- Participate in diverse activities and maintain social contacts
- Statements of adjustment to role reversal status and resolution of conflicts regarding care of client
- Ability to manage client's behavior changes and cognitive deficits

Cerebrovascular Accident

Cerebrovascular accident (stroke) is classified as either ischemic or hemorrhagic with the ischemic type more prevelant. Risk factors that predispose to stroke increase with age resulting in the greatest incidence of the disease in the elderly population. Manifestations of stroke, depending on the area of the brain affected, include neuromuscular deficits (paralysis, akinesia, decreased muscle tone and reflex activity, impaired integration of movements), communication deficits (aphasia, dysarthria), lack of affective control (exaggerated or unpredictable), intellectual impairment (memory, judgement, inability to learn), spacial-perceptual impairment (hemianopsmia, distance judgment, agnosia, apraxia, perception of self).

MEDICAL CARE

Anticoagulants: heparin IV or SC initially followed by warfarin (Coumadin) PO to reduce risk of further thrombus accumulation and to prevent recurrent clot formation by inhibiting prothrombin synthesis and reducing vitamin K dependent clotting factors

Platelet aggregation inhibitors: aspirin (ASA), dipyridamole (Persantine) PO to prevent clot formation and subsequent occlusion

Corticosteroids: prednisone (Deltasone) PO as an antinflammatory to reduce inflammatory reaction which increases intracranial pressure

Hyperosmotics: mannitol (Osmitrol) IV to reduce intracranial pressure caused by edema

Antihypertensives: (angeiotensin converting enzyme inhibitors, beta-adrenegic blockers, calcium channel blocker) PO alone or in combination to control blood pressure

Prothrombin (PT), activated partial thromboplastin time (APTT): Monitors anticoagulant therapy to reveal effectiveness of treatment

Skull x-ray: Reveals evidence of shift if hematoma or cerebral edema present

CT scan: Reveals cerebral edema, presence, extent and location of thrombus, embolus or hemorrhage

Brain nuclear scan: Reveals disruption in the blood-brain barrier, area of infarction, size and location of matoma

Magnetic resonance imaging: Reveals presence, extent and location of ischemia, edema, hemorrhage of brain

Electroencephalogram: Reveals brain's electrical activity at area of infarction or hemorrhage

Carotid endarterectomy: Surgical removal of atherosclerotic plaque from intima of carotid artery

NURSING CARE PLANS

Essential nursing diagnoses and plans associated with this condition:

Ineffective airway clearance (44)

Related to: Tracheobronchial obstruction from state of consciousness and potential for aspiration
Defining characteristics: Ineffective cough, tachypnea, dyspnea, abnormal breath sounds (crackles), change in rate, depth of respirations, decreased response to stimuli, choking, ineffective smallowing

Cerebrovascular Accident

←   Aging   →

↓   ↓   ↓   ↓

Hypertension   Artherosclerosis, transient ischemic attacks   Cardiac condition

↓   ↓   ↓

Cerebral hemorrhage   Thrombosis of cerebral vessel   Embolus originating in heart breaks away and enters circulation to cerebrum

↓

Cerebral infarction   ←

↓   ↓

Decreased flow of blood to area in brain affecting oxygen, nutrients, metabolic substances and removal of waste

↓

Cerebral edema, congesion in area

↓

←   Tissue compression and impaired function   →

↓   ↓   ↓

Anterior cerebral   Middle cerebral   Posterior cerebral

↓   ↓   ↓

Confusion   Arm paralysis   Hemiparesis
Impaired thought process   Hemianopia   Ataxia
Contralateral paresis or leg paralysis   Aphasia   Visual disturbances
Urinary incontinence   Agnosia   Dysphasia
Sensory deficits   Perceptual deficits   Dysphonia

↓   ↓   ↓

Return of tissue perfusion, reduced edema

↓

Cell survival and functional improvement

Altered tissue perfusion: cerebral (6)

Related to: interruption of arterial flow from infarct, hemorrhage
Defining characteristics: Confusion, changes in mentation, lethargy, stupor, coma, increased edema and cerebral pressure, headache, sensory, motor, cognitive, emotional dysfunction

Sensory/perceptual alterations: visual, tactile (72)

Related to: Altered sensory reception, transmission and/or integration from neurological disease or deficit
Defining characteristics: Change in visual acuity (hemiaosmia, diplopia, ptosis), loss of tactile perception in arm and/or leg (paresis, paralysis)

Impaired verbal communication (75)

Related to: Physical barrier from cerebral edema, necrosis of affected area
Defining characteristics: Aphasia, dysarthria, sensory deficits, impaired thought processes, difficulty speaking and writing, impaired comprehension, impaired articulation and phonation

Impaired physical mobility (196)

Related to: Neuromuscular impairment of paresis, paralysis
Defining characteristics: Leg and/or arm weakness or paralysis, muscle atrophy, flaccidity, deformity, contracture of affected limb(s), inability to purposefully move within physical environment

Altered nutrition: less than body requirements (118)

Related to: Inability to ingest food from dysphagia, absent gag reflex
Defining characteristics: Anorexia, choking, aspiration, inability to feed self, food remaining in mouth, weight loss, coma

Functional incontinence (154)

Related to: Sensory, cognitive or mobility deficits from stroke
Defining characteristics: Poor bladder control, incontinent episodes, unpredictable passage of urine

Constipation (121)

Related to: Less than adequate physical activity or immobility, dietary intake of bulk and neuromuscular impairment (paresis, dysphagia, paralysis)
Defining characteristics: Hard-formed stool, decreased bowel sounds, frequency less than usual pattern

Risk for impaired skin integrity (246)

Related to: External mechanical factor of pressure, shearing force
Defining characteristics: Paralysis, immobility, redness, warmth of an area

Sexual dysfunction (181)

Related to: Altered function, illness
Defining characteristics: Verbalization of problem, limitations imposed by illness, impotence, inability to achieve sexual satisfaction

SPECIFIC DIAGNOSES AND CARE PLANS

Unilateral neglect

Related to: Effects of disturbed perceptual abilities (hemiaosmia)
Defining characteristics: Consistent inattention to stimuli on affected side, does not look toward affected side, leaves food on plate on affected side

Outcome Criteria

Absence of safety hazards or injury to affected side.

Interventions	Rationales
Assess for safety hazards for client that ignores affected side	Removes potential for injury when unaware of injury threat
Utilize siderails, soft restraints or surveillance of positioning of affected side	Protects affected side from injury
Arrange articles in the environment for daily needs within perceptual field; follow by placing on affected side and encouraging to attend to affected side	Compensates for deficit
Assist to judge position and distance; assist with activities	Prepares for independence
Provide clear pathways, good lighting, eliminate small rugs	Prevents accidental falls

Interventions	Rationales
Continue reminding to turn head to affected and unaffected sides, rub and touch affected side frequently	Increases awareness of affected side

Information, Instruction, Demonstration

Interventions	Rationales
Provide instructions verbally and in small amounts, refer to affected side frequently	Promotes communication and understanding by client
Instruct to remind to care for affected side, perform daily exercises of affected side and to utilize affected limb when possible	Prevents neglect and deterioration of affected side

Discharge or Maintenance Evaluation

- Affected arm and/or leg without trauma or injury
- Affected arm and/or leg included in daily care

Ineffective individual coping

Related to: Multiple life changes (limitations imposed on lifestyle by stroke)
Defining characteristics: Inability to meet role expectations, inability to meet basic needs, chronic fatigue, alteration in societal participation

Related to: Inadequate coping method
Defining characteristics: Inability to problem-solve, inappropriate use of defense mechanisms, poor self-2 15Y

Outcome Criteria

Adaptation to chronic disabilities with optimal adjustments in lifestyle in relation to medical condition

Interventions	Rationales
Assess use of coping skills, ability to cope with fear associated with changes in physical/mental patterns and fatigue, chronicity of worry and anxiety	Older adults display outstanding ability to cope and adapt, although inability to maintain independence and control over life leads to frustration and negative feelings about life-style
Assist to identify positive defense mechanisms and promote their use; new behaviors to be learned	Use of defense mechanisms that have worked in past increases ability to cope and promotes self-esteem
Provide environment that allows for free expression of concerns and fears	Encourages trust and relieves anxiety

Information, Instruction, Demonstration

Interventions	Rationales
Social and coping skills with problem-solving approaches	Prevents disengagement and promotes coping ability with lifestyle changes
Relaxation techniques	Reduces anxiety and stress associated with decreasing functioning status
New ways or methods to adapt to new roles, to new situations or needs	Provides for alternatives and that increase participation independence in activities

Interventions	Rationales
Suggest psychotherapy or support groups if appropriate	Provides variety of techniques to reduce anxiety and stress

Discharge or Maintenance Evaluation

- Uses appropriate coping and problem-solving skills in adapting to functional losses
- Level of independence appropriate for functional ability
- Asks for assistance when needed
- Verbalizes reduced anxiety and fear
- Participates in social activities according to preference and activity tolerance

Knowledge deficit

Related to: Lack of exposure to information and cognitive limitations (medication regimen or rehabilitation))
Defining characteristics: Request for information, anxiety regarding potential errors

Outcome Criteria

Correct administration of medications and follow-up care to ensure safe dosages; optimal return of functional abilities

Interventions	Rationales
Assess orders for anticoagulant and antihypertensive therapy	Provides information of medication regimen in place for client
Inform of importance of having lab test done as prescribed	Ensures proper dosage or need for adjustment

Interventions	Rationales
Inform of reason for medication, action, dose, time to take, expected result and identification of side effects to report; involve family in instruction	Appropriate teaching enhances compliance and accurate administration of medications
Use teaching aids and written instructions for teaching	Promotes reinforcement of learning
Report any abnormal bleeding such as bruising, hematuria, bloody stools, petichiae; inform to use soft toothbrush, electric razor, avoid contact with sharp instruments	Side effect of anticoagulant therapy indicating dosage adjustment
Offer written schedule for physical, occupational speech therapy	Promotes rehabilitation of dysfunctional aspects of the disease

Discharge or Maintenance Evaluation

- Correct administration of medications and control of side effects
- Compliance in follow-up lab tests, reporting side effects

Neurosensory Deficits

Sensory deficits in the elderly population occur over long periods of time, affect more than one of the senses at the same time, are cumulative and result in sensory deprivation, overload and distortion. The increased incidence of diseases (diabetes, CVA, glaucoma, cataract) and health conditions (infections, vitamin deficiencies, dehydration, fever, trauma) increase the vulnerability of the older adult to sensory deprivation when compounded by the structural and functional changes in the system. The result is a decreased reception and perception of stimuli that leads to confusion, disorientation, difficulty concentrating and thinking, decreased intellectual activity and ability, anxiety, depression and mood swings. Sensory loss involves the senses affecting vision (cataract, glaucoma, macular degeneration, presbyopia), hearing (presbycusis), taste (hypogeusia), smell (dysosmia), and touch (somesthesia) and affect ability to express feelings and exchange experiences.

MEDICAL CARE

Otic anti-infectives, emulsants: carbamide peroxide (Debrox) ear application to facilitate cleansing by loosening excessive or impacted cerumen to prevent cerumenosis

Mydriatics: epinephrine (Epifrin) eye drops to produce dilation of pupils by blocking responses of iris and ciliary muscles to cholinergic stimulation, also decreases intraocular pressure

Miotics: pilocarpine (Pilocar) eye drops to reduce intraocular pressure by facilitating outflow of aqueous humor and reducing production of aqueous humor

Optic anti-infectives: bacitracin (Baciguent Ophthalmic) eye ointment to destroy microorganisms by interfering with cell wall synthesis

Cortico steroid: Prednisolone (Inflanase Forte) eye drops to suppression inflammatory process

Snellen test: Visual screening to reveal visual impairment

Audiology test: Screening to reveal hearing impairment, speech perception, tone acuity

Tonometry: Reveals intraocular pressure

Ophthalmoscope examination: Reveals cataract formation by revealing opacity

Otoscope examination: Reveals cerumen in the ear, presence of infection

Perimetry: Reveals peripheral vision and visual fields

Gonioscopy: Reveals anterior chamber for glaucoma and inflammation

Cataract extraction and lens insertion: Surgical treatment to remove and replace lens

Iridectomy: Establish a channel to filter the aqueous fluid

NURSING CARE PLANS

Essential nursing diagnoses and plans associated with these conditions:

Sensory/perceptual alterations: visual, auditory, kinesthetic, gustatory, tactile, olfactory (72)

Related to: Institutionalization, aging, chronic illness of dementia, atherosclerosis, diabetes mellitus, thyroid dysfunction

Glaucoma

Aging	Inflamation of uvea	Cataract surgery
↓	↓	↓
Enlarging lens Degenerative changes in aqueous outflow	Blockage of outflow channels	Poor wound healing Loss of aqueous humor
↓	↓	↓

Aging
↓
Enlarging lens
Degenerative changes
in aqueous outflow
↓

↓   Secondary glaucoma   Secondary glaucoma

Decreased drainage of aqueous
humor through canal of Schlemm   ↓
↓

Increased intraocular pressure   ↓
↓

Pressure on optic nerve
Nerve tissue ischemia   ↓
↓

Primary open-angle glaucoma   ↓
↓

→   Headaches, frequent change of glasses
Decreased peripheral vision
(tunnel vision)
Decreased night vision
Transient blurring vision
Haloes about lights
Decreased fields
↓

Blindness

Macular Degeneration

Aging/Senile degeneration

↓

Decreased nourishment of macular area by choroid (scelerosis of choriocapillaries)
New vessel development

↓

Detachment of macular area

↓

Loss of function of light sensitive cones

↓

Loss of central vision (dark or distorted)
Unimpaired peripheral vision

↓

Difficulty seeing at long distances
Difficulty in doing close work, reading
Difficulty in distinguishing colors
Difficulty in seeing faces clearly

↓

Blindness

Defining characteristics: Change in behavior patterns, disorientation, changes in cognitive abilities, changes in sensory perception

Related to: Altered sensory reception, transmission and/or integration from cataract, glaucoma, reduced perception of taste, smell, touch, degenerative sensory disorders of presbyopia, presbycusis, macular degeneration
Defining characteristics: Visual and auditory distortions, loss of interest and intake of food, apathy and reduced social interactions, inability to feel pain, pressure or temperature changes

Impaired verbal communication (75)

Related to: Decrease in circulation to brain from cerebrovascular accident
Defining characteristics: Disorientation, aphasia, dysarthia

Related to: Age related factors of cognitive or sensory deficits, neurological disease of Parkinson's, Alzheimer's
Defining characteristics: Does not or cannot speak, auditory deficit, impaired articulation, inability to find, name words, inability to identify objects, difficulty with phonation, stuttering, slurring

Risk for impaired skin integrity (246)

Related to: Internal factor of altered sensation (somesthesia)
Defining characteristics: Inability to feel pressure, inability to feel heat/cold, inability to feel pain

SPECIFIC DIAGNOSES AND CARE PLANS

Altered nutrition: less than body requirements

Related to: Inability to ingest food (hypoguesia, dysosmia)
Defining characteristics: Reduced dietary intake and meal enjoyment, lack of interest in food, reported altered taste and smell sensations

Outcome Criteria

Adequate nutritional intake with increased satisfaction with meals.

Interventions	Rationales
Assess ability to discriminate odors, flavors, food preferences	Determines extent of taste and smell deficit, loss of taste for sweet and salty flavors; loss of smell affects ability to taste and enjoy foods
Note tendency to add sugar to beverages, extra salt to food, ingestion of sweets	Indicates reduced taste perception which may result in weight gain or noncompliance with dietary restrictions
Offer mouth care before and after meals	Fresh, clean mouth promotes appetite, stimulates taste buds
Remove strong offensive odors	Interferes with appetite and interest in eating
Expose to strong pleasant odors of food cooking	Stimulates olfactory perception
Garnish and serve food in an attractive setting	Promotes appetite

Presbyopia

Aging

↓

Lens thicker and fiber becomes less elastic
Lens becomes larger and harder preventing flattening

↓

Decreased accommodation for near vision (farsightedness)
Lens yellowing and decreased opacity

↓

Range of focus diminished
Decreased peripheral vision
Decreased night vision
Blurred vision

↓

Progressive visual loss

↓

Holds objects at a distance
Withdrawal, social isolation
Disorientation, illusions

Presbycusis

Aging

↓

Sclerosis or atrophy of tympanic membrane
Loss of cells at base of cochlea
Excessive cerumen in middle ear

↓

Progressive bilateral symmetrical sensioneural hearing loss (transmission of sound to brain)

↓

Loss of hearing high frequency sounds and sibilant consonants (f, s, the, ch, sh)
Latter loss of consonants (b, t, p, k, d)
Sound distortion
Word dicrimination loss (phonetic regression)

↓

Unable to follow verbal direction/instruction
Withdrawal from conversaion
Speaks too loudly or softly
Difficulty understanding speech with frequent requests to repeat communication

Hypogensia, Dysosmia, Somethesia

Smoking/allergy	Aging	Neuropathy/circulatory insufficiency
↓	↓	↓
Hypogensia	Dysosmia	Somethesia
↓	↓	↓
Decreased number of taste buds/papilla	Reduction in ability to smell	Loss of tactile perception
↓	↓	↓
Loss of taste of sweet/ salty flavors	Inability to smell smoke Ability to discriminate strong odors	Inability to feel pain, heat/cold to skin
↓	↓	↓
Use of heavy seasoning Prefers sweet, salty foods Reduced dietary intake/ meal enjoyment	Safety hazard if warning devices not in use	Burns, trauma

Interventions	Rationales
Establish a regular meal time with a pleasant environment to join others at mealtime	Promotes interest and social opportunity during meals
Offer preferred foods of a proper texture and that can be picked up or eaten with assistive utensils	Promotes interest and desire to eat
Include foods with zinc from fruit and vegetable group	Promotes gustatory perception
Offer meals at times indicated by nutritional assessment or when hungry or requesting food	Following established pattern promotes successful food intake

Information, Instruction, Demonstration

Interventions	Rationales
Advise to eat at a table in sitting position and to feed self as much as possible	Promotes normal pattern of having meals
Plan menu to include cultural preferences, special dietary restrictions and appropriate consistency for ingestion	Promotes compliance to dietary regimen
Explain reason for decrease in gustatory and olfactory perception	Aging causes decreased number of taste buds and ability to discriminate odors

Discharge or Maintenance Evaluation

- Weight maintained within baseline level
- Statements of increased interest and appetite at mealtime
- Ingestion of adequate amounts of food from basic food groups

Risk for injury

Related to: Internal biochemical regulatory function (sensory dysfunction)
Defining characteristics: Poor visual acuity, poor auditory acuity, decreased kinesthetic perception, poor olfactory acuity, lack of safety education/precautions

Outcome Criteria

Trauma or injury prevented and safe environment established.

Interventions	Rationales
Assess degree of sensory loss and evolving conditions that affect ability to maintain safe lifestyle	In normal aging, there is a gradual loss in vision, hearing, smell, taste, touch
Encourage to wear prescribed hearing aid, corrective glasses depending on presence of condition	Increases or corrects problem to promote safety
Identify cues to presence of illusions in environment common to elderly	May lead to accidents if incorrect assumptions are made about objects, distance or space which are hazards
Provide proper lighting without glare appropriate to area and need, place switch near bed	Promotes vision at stairways, bathroom, pathways, close work, reading

Interventions	Rationales
Suggest Lifecare® alarm system	Form of warning system that brings assistance when activated
Use assistive aids when walking, telephone for the deaf	Provides support to prevent falls and call for help
Maintain clear pathways, dry floors, eliminate small rugs, wear good fitting slippers, provide hand bars in strategic areas	Prevents falls

Discharge or Maintenance Evaluation

- Environment free of safety hazards
- Assistive aids worn and warning devices installed and accepted
- Absence of injury

Information, Instruction, Demonstration

Interventions	Rationales
Importance of administration of eye medication	Promotes compliance to improve and maintain vision
Avoid night driving	Visual acuity decreased at night
Encourage bathing schedule, dating foods in refrigerator for proper disposal	May not be able to note offensive odors
Availability of pets that act as providers of assistance in presence of sensory deficits	Pets are trained to provide visual, auditory assistance

Parkinson's Disease

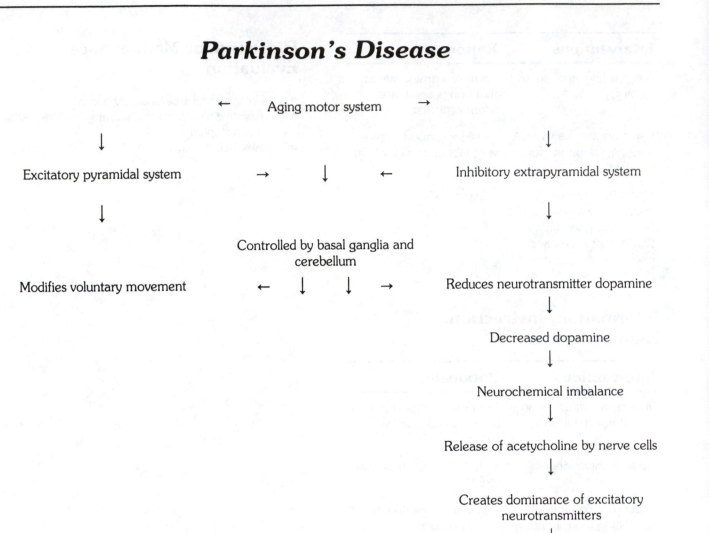

←   Aging motor system   →

↓   ↓

Excitatory pyramidal system   →   ↓   ←   Inhibitory extrapyramidal system

↓   ↓

Controlled by basal ganglia and
cerebellum

Modifies voluntary movement   ←   ↓   ↓   →   Reduces neurotransmitter dopamine

↓

Decreased dopamine

↓

Neurochemical imbalance

↓

Release of acetycholine by nerve cells

↓

Creates dominance of excitatory
neurotransmitters

↓

Muscle hypertonicity/rigidity
Tremor at rest
Kinesia

↓

Progression to total dependence

↓

Akinesia
Bowel, bladder dysfunction
Dysphasia
Poor articulation
Dyspnea
Depression

Parkinson's Disease

Parkinson's disease is a neurologic disorder that usually develops after the age of 50 and increases in incidence with age. It is a disorder of the basal ganglia of the extrapyramidal system which acts by modifying the pyramidal system which controls voluntary motor function. The disease is progressive and characterized by slowing and weakening movements, rigidity, and tremors until complete dependence occurs as the severity of symptoms increase. The neuromuscular and motor function changes eventually result in respiratory, elimination, mobility, and ingestion impairments.

MEDICAL CARE

Antiparkinsonians (dopamineragonist): carbidopa/levodopa (Sinemet) PO to inhibit metabolism of levodopa and permit more levodopa available for transport to the brain, bromocriptine (Parlodel) PO to activate dopamine receptors for relief of tremor, rigidity, kinesia

Anticholinergics: benzotropine (Cogentin) PO to treat tremors by reducing excess cholinergic effect associated with dopamine deficiency

Monoamine oxidase inhilutor: selegilene (Eldepryl) PO to augment the effect of dopamine by inhibiting the enzyme that degrades it

NURSING CARE PLANS

Essential nursing diagnoses and plans associated with this condition:

Ineffective airway clearance (44)

Related to: Tracheobronchial obstruction, infection from aspiration, truncal rigidity
Defining characteristics: Dysphagia, inability to cough, dyspnea, tachypnea, diminished breath sounds, crackles, changes in rate and depth of respirations

Altered thought processes (70)

Related to: Physiological changes from medication regimen
Defining characteristics: Cognitive dissonance, memory loss, confusion, depression, argumentative, impaired ability to reason, make decisions, grasp ideas, maintain attention, toxic blood level of medication, akinesia (levodopa)

Impaired verbal communication (75)

Related to: Physical barrier from hypertonicity and rigidity of facial muscles
Defining characteristics: Cannot speak, impaired articulation, slurring, slow monotonous speech, drooling saliva, repetitive speech, rapid speech, high-pitched, hoarse, trembling speech

Impaired physical mobility (196)

Related to: Neuromuscular impairment of tremors, rigidity, bradykinesia
Defining characteristics: Inability to purposefully move within physical environment, slow involuntary movements, spontaneous movement (jerky actions), postural and gait disturbance, small, shuffling steps, leaning forward with head bent, uncontrollable gait with difficulty starting and stopping when walking progression to akinesia

Altered nutrition: less than body requirements (118)

Related to: Inability to ingest food
Defining characteristics: Dysphagia, choking, coughing, rigidity of facial muscles

SPECIFIC DIAGNOSES AND CARE PLANS

Impaired swallowing

Related to: Neuromuscular impairment (dysphagia)
Defining characteristics: Stasis of food in oral cavity, slow eating, difficulty in swallowing, chewing, stiff, masklike face, choking, drooling, weight loss

Outcome Criteria

Adequate nutritional intake associated with minimal chewing and swallowing impairment. Minimal difficulty swallowing and management of food ingestion; absence of drooling.

Interventions	Rationales
Assess ability to chew, move food in mouth, swallow, presence of gag reflex, choking on food when eating	Stiff, rigid face muscles cause difficulty in eating and managing secretions in mouth
Assess adequacy of food intake, weight loss	Bradykinesia and uncompensated rigidity cause inability to ingest needed caloric intake
Allow time for eating and to take small amounts to chew	Slow movements require more time to prevent choking

Interventions	Rationales
Serve soft foods instead of liquids or purees; frequent high protein and caloric meals preferred	Easier to manipulate in mouth and swallow; provides essential nutrients
Offer candy or chewing gum; avoid bending head to maintain secretions in back of throat	Reminds to swallow to prevent drooling
Massage face and neck muscles	Assists to relax muscles before eating
Provide tissues or wipe mouth when needed	Removes drooling or food

Information, Instruction, Demonstration

Interventions	Rationales
Instruct in tongue movements to back of mouth	Assists in swallowing
Avoid speaking when eating	May encourage choking, prevent management of food in mouth
Use of assistive device for eating if appropriate	Promotes independence and control over mealtime, taking the time needed and bite size that can be managed
Diet selections that are soft, contain fiber if possible	Provides adequate nutrition and fiber for bowel elimination
Refer to occupational therapist	Provides self-feeding techniques

Discharge or Maintenance Evaluation

- Drooling managed and reduced, if possible
- Chews and swallows small amounts of food at a time
- Uses feeding device correctly
- Maintains fluid intake of 2 L/day and regular bowel elimination routine
- Practices tongue movement and manages food without choking

Risk for injury

Related to: Internal physical factor of altered mobility (bradykinesia, akinesia)
Defining characteristics: Involuntary movements, loss of postural adjustment (stooped causing imbalance), loss of arm swinging movement, difficulty initiating movement, shuffling gait (festination), slowness of movement, orthostatic hypotension, activity intolerance

Outcome Criteria

Absence of accidents or falls when ambulating.

Interventions	Rationales
Assess ability to walk, execution of movements, presence of spontaneous movements, fatigue level during activity	Result of physical and chemical alteration in the basic ganglia and structures in the extra-pyramidal system of CNS
Clear pathways, remove small rugs and furniture, provide lighting	Prevents falls and frustration when unable to step over any obstacle
Provide assistive aid for walking if appropriate	Promotes steadiness
Suggest walking with head up and body straight as possible	Prevents imbalance caused by posture, flexing knees and hips

Interventions	Rationales
Allow time to accomplish tasks, walking, rising from lying position or sitting position	Promotes activity and self-esteem when independence is encouraged; movements are slow and must be consciously willed before accomplished

Information, Instruction, Demonstration

Interventions	Rationales
Instruct in methods to turn and walk slowly raising toes before taking a step and putting heels down first to follow through with step, turn by walking instead of crossing feet	Provides balanced gait for ambulation and turning when shuffling, small steps and involuntary movements are present
Inform to roll to side in bed and sit up for a period of time and dangle feet before rising to standing position	Prevents orthostatic hypotension effects of dizziness and faintness

Discharge or Maintenance Evaluation

- Ambulation without falls
- Use of walking aids correctly
- Modifies walking and turning without falling
- Maintains environment free of safety hazards

Ineffective individual coping

Related to: Multiple life changes (progressive chronic disease and associated limitations)
Defining characteristics: Inability to manage stressors, inability to meet basic needs (ADL), change in communication patterns, alteration in societal partici-

pation, lack of appetite, poor self-esteem, depression, insomnia

Outcome Criteria

Increased ability to cope with deteriorating condition.

Interventions	Rationales
Assess feelings of increasing loss of control, body image, social isolation, presence of anxiety, depression, acceptance of disabilities	Emotional adjustment difficult and results in multiple socio-psychological problems as increasing dependence becomes apparent
Assist to identify needs and establish goals that fit stage of disease	Promotes control and decision-making which increases self-esteem
Provide calm, nonjudgemental environment for expression of feelings and concerns	Promotes trust and reduces anxiety
Offer diversional activities appropriate to requests and level of intelligence; promote positive and stimulating activities, family/client reminiscence	Intelligence and cognitive abilities remain intact
Encourage independence in ADL within functional limitations	Permits maximal control over care needs and prevents frustration

Information, Instruction, Demonstration

Interventions	Rationales
Inform that engaging in social activities will provide diversion and mobility	Prevents isolation, depression and promotes coping with physical changes

Interventions	Rationales
Refer to counseling or social worker as appropriate	Offers encouragement and suggestions for relaxation and coping with changes
Suggest day care, support groups	Provides information and social interaction increasing knowledge of disease and support from those with similar problems

Discharge or Maintenance Evaluation

- Level of social and self-care activities appropriate for functional ability
- Statements that ability to cope with changes increasing as assistance or independence maintained
- Achieves self-derived goals for reducing anxiety (relaxation techniques) and improving self-esteem (control and independence)

Sleep Disorders

The most common sleep disorders found in the elderly population are insomnia and sleep apnea. Other disorders include hypersomia or excessive sleep and nocturnal behavior or Sundowner's Syndrome that is manifested by disorientation and wandering during the late afternoon and evening time frames. Sleep needs of the elderly may be the same as in other stages of adulthood or slightly less and are often a concern because sleep patterns change with age. Insomnia is characterized by inability or difficulty in falling asleep, frequent awakenings during sleep, awakening early in the morning. Depending on individual perception, some elderly feel that they have not slept when, in actuality, evidence suggests that they have slept. Sleep apnea is characterized by cessation of breathing for periods of time during sleep, causing decreased oxygen concentration which wakes client before completing REM sleep phase. This results in sleepiness, lethargy and exhaustion and has been associated with sudden death and dysrhythmias in the elderly. Hypersomia is characterized by fatigue, blackouts, memory problems, hallucinations, and nocturnal behaviors such as talking, screaming, moaning, scratching, coughing, and teeth grinding.

MEDICAL CARE

Sedatives/Hypnotics (benzodiazepines): triazolam (Halicon), temazepam (Restoril) PO for short-term relief of insomnia

Sedative/Hyponotic (Barbiturates): amobarbital (Sodium Amytal) PO to treat disrupted sleep cycles in dementia conditions

Antidepressants: protriptyline (Triptil) PO to reduce apneic episodes

Respiratory stimulants: methylphenidate (Ritalin) PO to increase respiratory drive in central apnea

Electroencephalogram: Reveals sleep stages

Electrooculogram: Reveals sleep stages

Sleep lab testing: Overnight monitoring of sleep to reveal cerebral, muscle, rib cage, abdominal and eye movements, nasal airflow, oxygen saturation and electrical activity of heart

Impedance pneumography: Reveals respiratory effort

NURSING CARE PLANS

Essential nursing diagnoses and plans associated with these conditions:

Ineffective breathing pattern (44)

Related to: Tracheobronchial obstruction of sleep apnea
Defining characteristic: Snoring, cessation of breathing for periods of time, hypoxia, fatigue, yawning, lethargy

Altered thought processes (70)

Related to: Sleep deprivation from insomnia or sleep apnea
Defining characteristics: Confusion, disorientation, memory changes, lethargy, cognitive dissonance

Sleep pattern disturbance (77)

Related to: Internal factor of illness (heart, renal, thyroid)

Insomnia

Aging	Depression	Leg Cramps	Hyperthyroidism	Electrolyte imbalance
↓	Boredom	Pain	Heart failure	Hypoglycemia
			Renal insufficiency	Drug reaction
Decreased stages III	↓	↓	↓	Alcohol toxicity
and IV (deep sleep)				Liver failure
↓				↓

Confusion/dimentia

↓

Exaggerated confu-
sion at night

↓

Wandering
Sleeplessness

→   Insomnia   ←
                              ↓

More frequent wakenings at night
Decreased intensity of sleep
↓

Spends more time in bed but feels tired
Naps during day
Fatigue, irritability, lethargy
Disorientation
Difficulty falling asleep
Awakening early in morning

Sleep Apnea

Obesity   Alcohol   Central nervous   Aging   Central nervous
                                  system depressants   system disorders

                                                                                 ↓

                                                                          Encephalitis
                                                                          Brain stem infarction
   ↓   ↓   ↓   ↓   Bulbar poliomyelitis

                                                                                 ↓

                  Obstruction of upper airway   Respiratory drive
                                                                               cease

                                                                                 ↓

                                                                          Absence of move-
                           ↓   ment of chest or
                                                                          abdomen muscles

                                                                                 ↓

              Obstructive apnea   → Mixed apnea ←   Central apnea
                           ↓   ↓

          Loud snoring interrupted by
             periods of silence   Awakening during
          Cessation of breathing   night
             for periods of time   Fatigue
             Sleep walking   Depression
             Morning headache   Sexual dysfunction
             Sleepiness during day
             Lethargy, yawning
          Sexual dysfunction (impotence)

                           ↓

          Cardiac arrhythmias
             Polycythemia
          Systemic/pulmonary hypertension
             Hypoxemia

Defining characteristics: Interrupted sleep, difficulty falling asleep, awakening early, fatigue, lethargy, irritability, disorientation, complaints of not feeling rested

Related to: Psychological stress (depression, confusion, boredom)
Defining characteristics: Insomnia, sleeplessness, naps during day, fatigue, lethargy, disorientation, expressionless face

Related to: External factor of environmental changes (stimuli, obstructive sleep apnea)
Defining characteristics: Interrupted sleep, exhaustion, snoring, long periods of silence, cessation of breathing, sleepiness during day, yawning, lethargy, morning headache, loss of libido

SPECIFIC DIAGNOSES AND CARE PLANS

Anxiety

Related to: Threat to change in health status (sleep deprivation interfering with sense of well-being)
Defining characteristics: Communication of feeling exhaustion, insomnia, sleep apnea, communication of fear of consequences of sleep apnea

Related to: Change in role functioning (sexual dysfunction, decreased energy compounded by exhaustion)
Defining characteristics: Communication of increased tension, feelings of inadequacy, uncertainty, impotence, depression, sleep apnea, insomnia

Outcome Criteria

Reduced anxiety level as sleep deprivation resolved.

Interventions	Rationales
Assess anxiety level, depression, feelings about results of sleep disorder and effect on lifestyle and function	Persistent sleep loss that results in mental, physical and sexual dysfunction causes threat to health and anxiety which in turn results in continued sleeplessness
Provide calm, supportive environment, avoid stimuli	Reduces anxiety and promotes trust
Provide relaxation exercises, guided imagery, music	Reduces anxiety by distraction
Listen to expressions of concern; discuss sexual concerns if willing	Allows for venting of feelings and control of environment
Respond positively to complaints and requests without expressing disappointment or judgments	Promotes trusting relationship

Information, Instruction, Demonstration

Interventions	Rationales
Potential for continued sleeplessness if anxiety level high	Creates chronic sleep problem and difficulty resolving insomnia
Types of relaxation techniques that assist to reduce anxiety	Allows for preferred selection for compliance and control over decision making
Return of sexual satisfaction when sleep adequate	Temporary condition related to sleep apnea

Discharge or Maintenance Evaluation

- Communication that anxiety reduced and manageable
- Communication of belief that health and sexual function will not be compromised after resolution of sleep problem

Transient Ischemic Attack

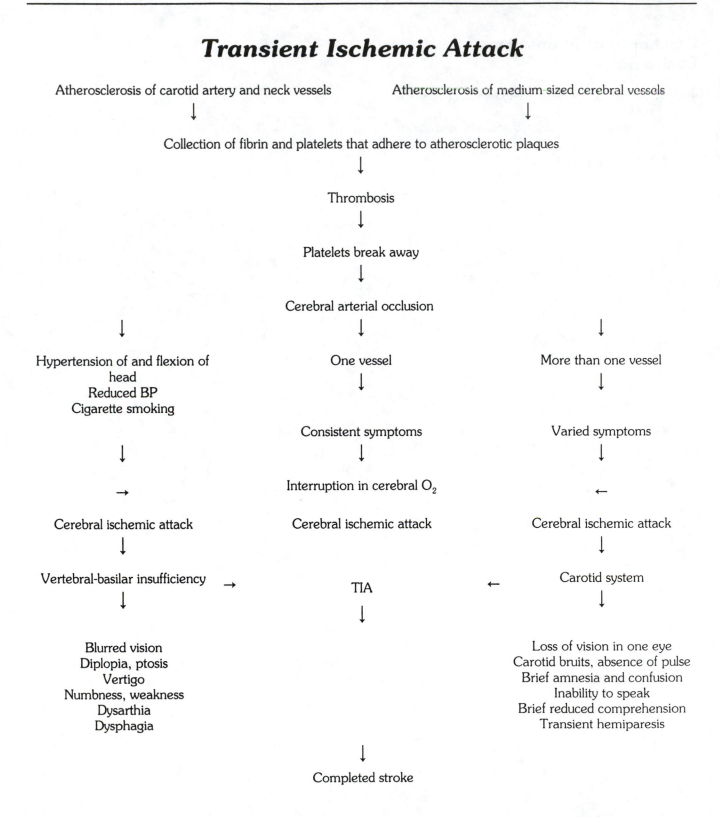

Atherosclerosis of carotid artery and neck vessels   Atherosclerosis of medium-sized cerebral vessels

↓   ↓

Collection of fibrin and platelets that adhere to atherosclerotic plaques

↓

Thrombosis

↓

Platelets break away

↓

Cerebral arterial occlusion

↓

Hypertension of and flexion of head Reduced BP Cigarette smoking	One vessel ↓	More than one vessel ↓

↓   Consistent symptoms   Varied symptoms

↓   ↓   ↓

→   Interruption in cerebral O_2 ←

Cerebral ischemic attack   Cerebral ischemic attack   Cerebral ischemic attack

↓   ↓

Vertebral-basilar insufficiency → TIA ← Carotid system

↓   ↓   ↓

Blurred vision
Diplopia, ptosis
Vertigo
Numbness, weakness
Dysarthia
Dysphagia

Loss of vision in one eye
Carotid bruits, absence of pulse
Brief amnesia and confusion
Inability to speak
Brief reduced comprehension
Transient hemiparesis

↓

Completed stroke

Transient Ischemic Attack

A brief, temporary episode of neurologic loss of vision, motor and/or sensory function that may last from a few minutes to 24 hours. Sometimes referred to as "little strokes"; only about one-third of those experiencing TIAs go on to have completed strokes. They are caused by an interruption of blood flow to the brain and are associated with conditions such as hypertension, atherosclerosis, hyperlipidemia and polycythemia in the elderly population.

MEDICAL CARE

Platelet aggregation inhibitors: dipyridamole (Persantine) alone or with aspirin (Bayer) PO to prevent platelet aggregation at atherosclerotic plaque site

Anticoagulants: warfarin (Coumadin) PO to inhibit prothrombin synthesis and decrease clotting potential

Carotid Doppler studies: Auscultates, visualizes, photographs carotid bruits

Carotid, cerebral angiography: Reveals intracranial and cervical vessels and blood flow

Oculoplethysmography: Reveals and measures blood flow through ophthalmic artery

Carotid endarterectomy: Surgical removal of atherosclerotic plaque from carotid artery

Lipid panel: Reveals lipoproteins, cholesterol and triglyceride level and relationship to atherosclerosis and potential for risk factors

NURSING CARE PLANS

Essential nursing diagnoses and plans associated with this condition:

Altered tissue perfusion: cerebral (6)

Related to: Interruption of arterial flow from atherosclerosis
Defining characteristics: Changes in carotid pulse, carotid bruits, confusion, changes in mentation, vertigo, changes in vision, numbness, weakness, inability to speak, amnesia

Risk for trauma (198)

Related to: Internal factors (weakness, poor vision, balancing difficulties, cognitive difficulties)
Defining characteristics: Dizziness, headache, blurred vision, diplopia, transient hemiparesis anemia, confusion, lack of safety precautions

Altered thought processes (70)

Related to: Physiological changes from interruption of cerebral O_2
Defining characteristics: Confusion, vertigo, brief amnesia, decreased comprehension, memory deficit

Sensory-perceptual alteration: visual (72)

Related to: Altered status of sense organs from cerebral ischemic attacks

Defining characteristics: Blurred vision, diplopia, loss of vision in one eye, disoriented

SPECIFIC DIAGNOSES AND CARE PLANS

Knowledge deficit

Related to: Lack of information (medication and safety measures)
Defining characteristics: Request for information

Outcome criteria

Correct administration of medications and understanding of treatment plan.

Interventions	Rationales
Assess for knowledge of disease, and treatment regimen, prevention of complications	Provides information to plan teaching program
Wear cervical collar, avoid hyperextension, lateral movement of neck; any quick movements or position changes, rising from bed quickly	Compression on neck resulting from cervical vertebral changes may lead to symptoms of TIA or bradycardia; sudden position changes lead to dizziness
Proper administration of medications, why given and expected results, side effects and when to report them	Promotes compliance and desired effects of medications
Signs and symptoms of TIA activity to report to physician especially if lasts longer than 30 minutes	Prevents stroke; opportunity to adjust medications

Interventions	Rationales
Methods to hold on to furniture, use aids for walking, looking straight ahead when walking	Prevents falls during TIA
Method of rolling out of bed, rising from chair slowly	Prevents orthostatic hypotension

Discharge or Maintenance Evaluation

- Statements of signs and symptoms and treatment of TIA
- Performs safety measures when walking to prevent falls
- Correct adminsitration of medication regimen; reports adverse effects
- Takes measures to prevent attack and BP changes
- Reports TIA and visits physician for monitoring as prescribed
- Modifies environment to minimize safety hazards (hand bars, cane, chairs to sit on)

Gastrointestinal System

Gastrointestinal System

Alterations in the digestive process affected by the aging process include changes in secretion, reduction of nutrients, absorption, transport or motility. Nervous system changes also contribute to control organic functions by sensory and motor losses which affect peripheral nerve conduction, parasympathetic and sympathetic functions which affect intestinal motility and enzymatic release, and decreased vasomotor response which affects ingestion. A major number of complaints made by the elderly involve the gastrointestinal system beginning with the mouth and ending with the process of bowel elimination. The risk for digestive disorders are brought about from obstructive processes, absorption problems, vascular abnormalities and neurological changes in the aged population.

GENERAL GASTROINTESTINAL CHANGES ASSOCIATED WITH THE AGING PROCESS

Organ structure/anatomy

- Teeth enamel thins causing teeth to become brittle
- Grinding surface of teeth wears down causing a decreased force in biting and chewing
- Bone loss in oral structures causing difficulty in fitting dentures, chewing food and decreasing tooth support
- Thinning and drying of oral epithelium causing easily irritated and damaged mucous membranes
- Increasing body fat and decreasing lean body mass with changes in fat distribution or decreases in extremities and increases in abdomen and hips
- Gradual weight decreases with women, decreases slower than men
- Decreased subcutaneous tissue causing difficulty in environmental temperature adjustment
- Decrease in liver size; pancreatic atrophy causing a decrease in exocrine cells for enzyme production
- Alveolar degeneration and obstruction of the ducts of the pancreas causing blockage of secretions
- Decreased mucosal surface area of small intestines causing altered absorption of nutrients
- Atrophy of mucosa, muscle layers, arteriolar sclerosis, delay in peripheral nerve transmission of colon causing constipation or fecal incontinence
- Weakness of abdominal and pelvic muscles causing difficulty in defecation

Physiologic function

- Reduced saliva production causing dry mouth and potential for breakdown of oral mucosa
- Reduced number of taste buds causing altered taste and reduced food intake
- Change in pH of saliva from acidic to alkalinic causing increased tendency for tooth decay
- Decreased gag reflex causing swallowing difficulty
- Decreased peristaltic activity and relaxation of smooth muscle of lower esophagus causing delayed emptying, dilitation and reflux
- Decreased pepsin, hydrochloric acid secretion, intrinsic factor by stomach with a thinner mucosa and atrophic changes causing reduced absorption of vitamins B_1, B_2, B_{12}
- Reduced ptyalin with reduced saliva and reduced lipase and mucin secretion by stomach causing slowing of digestive process
- Decreased metabolic rate causing weight gain

- Decreased hepatic enzyme concentration causing a reduced enzyme response to drug metabolism and detoxification
- Bile thicker, contains higher cholesterol concentration and reduced in volume with emptying more difficult causing biliary tract disease (cholelithiasis) and obstruction with a decrease in fat soluble vitamin absorption by bile
- Decreased secretion of amylase, lipase and trypsin by pancreas causing impaired digestion of lipids and splitting of large polypeptides into peptides which are acted upon in a singular fashion by the small intestine
- Decreased absorption of nutrients by small intestine and reduced transport mechanism efficiency
- Decreased enzyme secretion causing increased time required for digestion and reduced bacterial flora in large intestine
- Decreased bowel motility, gastrocolic reflex, voluntary contraction of the external sphincter, amount of feces which all contribute to constipation or fecal incontinence
- Vasculature of digestive tract (artherosclerosis) causing decreased blood supply of nutrients to bowel and possibly tissue injury

ESSENTIAL NURSING DIAGNOSES AND CARE PLANS

Altered nutrition: less than body requirements

Related to: Inability to ingest or digest food or absorb nutrients because of biological or psychological factors

Defining characteristics: Body weight 20% or more under ideal for height and frame, reported inadequate food intake, weakness of muscles required for swallowing or mastication, lack of interest in food, reported altered taste/smell sensation, satiety immediately after ingesting food, abdominal pain or discomfort, sore, inflamed buccal cavity, depression, anxiety, social isolation, difficulty in feeding self, changes in mentation

Outcome Criteria

Adequate intake of appropriate nutrients with optimal weight for age, height and frame maintained.

Interventions	Rationales
Assess presence of anorexia, nausea, vomiting, dyspepsia, dysphagia, potential for choking or aspiration, fatigue, dyspnea	Provides information regarding factors associated with reduced intake of nutrients; lack of activity in the elderly contributes to anorexia
Assess usual eating pattern, ability to feed self, presence of cough and gag reflex, presence of cognitive deficits	Provides information for dietary planning
Assess condition of mouth and teeth, fit of dentures, food left in mouth	Provides ability to chew foods without discomfort
Assess weight every week on same scale at same time	Provides gain or loss information
Assess for caloric need for size and frame: likes and dislikes; 24 hour food intake analysis for calories and nutritional content	Determines need for dietary adjustments (inclusions or removal of foods); deficiencies result from type of foods eaten rather than amount of food eaten
Review side effects and food interactions of medications being taken	Some medications impair nutritional intake
Assess effort needed for essential physical functions and energy and endurance level	Fatigue impairs ability to chew and swallow foods
Offer diet of 6 small meals/day with high protein, carbohydrate foods that are easily chewed and swallowed	Maintains nutrition while preventing further muscle wasting

Interventions	Rationales
Offer high caloric liquid or custard supplements (Ensure)	Provides additional protein and caloric intake
Administer vitamin/ mineral supplement	Ensures adequate vitamin inclusion in diet for proper body function which can remain the same through life
Place in upright position for meals and remain in this position for 30 minutes	Prevents aspiration and promotes movement of food by gravity and peristalsis
Provide rest period, give oral care before and after meals; perform any treatments before meals	Enhances appetite and reduces difficulty in eating if dyspnea or reflux present
Crush oral medications and mix with food or request liquid form	Prevents choking and aspiration
Provide assistance with eating or allow time for self-feeding without rushing	Promotes independence and adequate intake without choking
If fluids hard to manipulate, blend fruits with water	Thicker substances are easier to swallow
Provide nutritionist for meal planning, especially if on a special diet	Promotes counseling that emphasizes behavior modification to ensure adequate nutritional intake
If unable to ingest food by mouth, administer tube feedings: • Warm feedings to room temperature • Aspirate tube to ensure patency • Aspirate stomach contents to assess for residual to prevent distention and vomiting	Alternate method of providing nutrients

Interventions	Rationales
• Retain upright position for 30 minutes after intermittent feedings; if feeding continuously, maintain position to prevent aspiration • Instill 30 ml water after feeding to clear tube • Utilize enteral infusion pump to regulate drop rate • Check bowel sounds after each feeding to ensure feeding tolerance • Maintain suctioning equipment at hand during feedings to remove feedings if choking or aspiration occurs	

Information, Instruction, Demonstration

Interventions	Rationales
Menu planning that includes basic 5 groups and proper distribution of protein (10-15%), carbohydrate (50-55%), fats (25-30% excluding animal fats) and with the necessary caloric content	Provides complete nutritional requirements with consideration for cultural preferences
Schedule meals as part of an activity schedule	Allows for meals without increased exertion or fatigue
Avoid intake of large amounts of food at one meal; have snacks available	Prevents nausea, overdistention, dyspepsia and upward pressure on diaphragm

Interventions	Rationales
Instruct to place food in back of mouth	Facilitates swallowing
Instruct in use of assistive aids (large-handled cups, straws, large-handled utensils, movable spoons)	Promotes self-feeding and independence
Report consistent weight loss	Indicates nutritional deficit
Instruct in special dietary requirements, disease dependent; make minimal changes if possible to maintain health in presence of disease	Promotes adequate nutrition without creating additional gastrointestinal or other system complications
Suggest eating with friend or companion as preferred; use TV or radio during meals	Promotes enjoyment of meal time and prevents isolation

Discharge or Maintenance Evaluation

- Stabilized body weight
- Daily intake of calculated calories and vitamin supplement
- Compliance with special dietary requirements
- Statement reflecting knowledge of daily requirements and proper nutrition for size and body frame
- Statements that appetite improved and meal schedule satisfactory
- Absence of mouth soreness, poor fitting dentures, toothache
- Absence of aspiration of food

Altered nutrition: more than body requirements

Related to: Excessive intake in relationship to metabolic need

Defining characteristics: Weight 10% over ideal for height and frame, sedentary activity level, increased food intake with decreased metabolic rate, high caloric snacks in addition to meals, pairing food with other activities, eating in response to social situations or anxiety, depression, boredom

Outcome Criteria

Return to baseline weight according to standards for size and frame.

Interventions	Rationales
Assess dietary history intake, eating patterns, importance of eating, where excesses can be limited	Provides information regarding factors associated with overweight or obesity problem; elderly tend to gain weight easily because of decreased activity and a lower metabolic rate
Assess amount of weight loss needed for body size, frame	Provides basis for dietary planning
Assess weight every week on same scale at same time	Provides goal achievement weight loss information
Assist to plan for realistic weekly goals for weight loss of 1 lb	Prevents frustration from not achieving goals
Provide schedule of activities that are not associated with meals or snacks	Utilizes calories and provides diversion from eating
Praise for successes and efforts to lose weight	Encourages continued progress

Information, Instruction, Demonstration

Interventions	Rationales
Offer menus and instruct in low caloric food selection that includes adequate nutritional intake	Promotes weight reduction program to follow
Keep a log of intake (type and amount) for analysis	Ensures adequate nutritional intake and caloric reduction
Suggest joining weight reduction program or community support group	Provides support for weight loss and behavior modification for reduced food intake

Discharge or Maintenance Evaluation

- Weight loss of 1 lb/week until stable
- Return to and maintenance of baseline weight
- Adequate nutritional intake with reduced calories
- Elimination of high caloric foods, fad diets during reduction program

Constipation

Related to: Less than adequate dietary intake and bulk (soft diet)
Defining characteristics: Frequency less than usual pattern, hard-formed stool, decreased bowel sounds, less than usual amount of stool, palpable mass, reported feeling of rectal fullness, abdominal pressure, inability to chew and swallow foods containing bulk, cellulose

Related to: Less than adequate physical activity (immobility)
Defining characteristics: Imposed bedrest, impaired physical mobility

Related to: Chronic use of medication and enemas
Defining characteristics: Use of laxatives, frequent bouts of constipation

Related to: Neuromuscular impairment (neurological disease)
Defining characteristics: Decreased bowel sounds, impaired peristalsis, lack of awareness of defecation urge

Related to: Weak abdominal musculature
Defining characteristics: Unable to expel stool, straining at stool, incomplete stool elimination, general weakness and fatigue

Related to: Emotional status (neurological/psychological conditions)
Defining characteristics: Confusion, agitation, cognitive deficit, lethargy, apathy, appetite impairment, depression

Related to: Musculoskeletal impairment (musculoskeletal disorders)
Defining characteristics: Immobility, fracture with cast/traction, unable to use commode/toilet, activity intolerance, weakness, pain, discomfort

Outcome Criteria

Soft formed stool elimination without effort maintained based on baseline pattern.

Interventions	Rationales
Assess bowel elimination pattern, daily habits, ability to sense and communicate urge to defecate, presence of anorexia, nausea, headache, painful hemorrhoids, history of constipation	Provides basis for establishing and maintaining bowel training program and reasons for inability or desire to defecate
Assess stool frequency and characteristics, abdominal distention and discomfort, presence of flatulence and straining at stool	Indicates constipation problem common in the elderly because of decreased motility and gastrocolic reflex causing stool to remain in colon longer and water to be reabsorbed

Interventions	Rationales
Assess mental and emotional state including LOC	Cognitive deficit and confusion affects awareness to defecate (feeling of distended rectum); emotional factors affect the desire and energy to defecate
Assess use of laxatives and/or enemas, other medications that may cause constipation	Perceived bowel expectations may be unrealistic and elderly often resort to laxative dependence for regularity which predisposes to constipation
Administer bulk laxative or stool softener until regular pattern is established	Promotes elimination of soft formed stool with increased motility for easier passage
Provide fluid intake of at least 2 L/day	Promotes greater fluid content of stool for easier passage
Provide diet that includes bulk if able to chew and swallow	Bulk degradation in colon assists in formation and passage of stool
Place on bedpan with bed raised or assist to commode or bathroom when request made to defecate	Promotes elimination when urge is present
Allow for privacy during elimination; return promptly when called	Elderly prize their privacy and consideration enhances elimination and comfort level
Institute bowel training program: • Maintain dietary and fluid requirements • Offer bedpan or bathroom 30 minutes after breakfast each day • Administer glycerin suppository 30 minutes before	Promotes regular bowel regimen

Interventions	Rationales
elimination if needed to encourage elimination until pattern established • Maintain consistency in schedule and approach	

Information, Instruction, Demonstration

Interventions	Rationales
Suggest avoiding caffeine-containing drinks and use of enemas	Diuretic effect causes loss of needed fluids
Suggest addition of prunes or prune juice to diet	Contains fiber and promotes peristalsis
Maintain activity or exercise schedule	Promotes propulsive bowel action

Discharge or Maintenance Evaluation

- Regular bowel elimination pattern established
- Stool soft and formed, expelled without cramping, straining
- Adjustments of fiber and fluid additions made for dietary intake
- Daily exercise regimen maintained within limitations
- Absence of fecal impaction or incontinence

Diarrhea

Related to: Dietary intake (soft, low residue diet)
Defining characteristics: Increased frequency, increased bowel sounds, loose, liquid stools, fluid/electrolyte imbalance, cramping, urgency, fecal incontinence

Related to: Medications (laxatives, antibiotics, chemotherapy)
Defining characteristics: Frequent passage of stools, loose, liquid or watery stools, abdominal pain, cramping

Related to: Inflammation, irritation, or malabsorption of bowel (gastrointestinal disorders)
Defining characteristics: Increased frequency of loose, liquid stools, cramping, increased bowel sounds, changes in color of stool, fever, malaise, blood, mucus, fatty substances in stool

Related to: Radiation (cancer therapy)
Defining characteristics: Increased frequency of loose, liquid stools, cramping, urgency, increased bowel sound

Outcome Criteria

Soft formed stool elimination based on baseline pattern.

Interventions	Rationales
Assess presence of diarrhea and characteristics, fecal impaction or incontinence, I&O if diarrhea severe	Diarrhea depletes fluids and electrolytes and results in weakness over an extended episode; liquid stool may pass around impaction and be expelled as diarrhea
Administer antidiarrheals	Decreases motility and controls number of bowel eliminations
Provide cleansing of anal area with mild soap and water, dry gently and well after each bowel movement	Prevents skin irritation from frequent eliminations
Provide skin ointment such as Nupercaine to anal area	Promotes comfort and protects from irritation
Collect stool specimen for lab examination (culture, toxins)	Reveals presence of toxins, bacterial infection of bowel

Interventions	Rationales
Maintain close proximity to commode, bathroom	Prevents embarrassing accidents

Information, Instruction, Demonstration

Interventions	Rationales
Comply with fluid and dietary inclusion as appropriate	Provides bulk to stool and fluid replacement
Inform that antibiotic regimens may result in diarrheal episode	Causes overgrowth infection resulting diarrhea as needed intestinal bacteria are destroyed
Avoid caffeine drinks, spicy foods, nuts, seeds, raw foods, flatulence-increasing foods such as cabbage, beans or onions	Acts as diuretic and increases fluid in colon; may be irritating to bowel and increase motility
Inform to avoid laxative use and mineral oil	Regular use compounds problem by creating dependency and interfering with normal elimination reflexes and mechanisms; mineral oil tends to be lost through sphincter and cause soiling and interferes with metabolism of fat-soluble vitamins

Discharge or Maintenance Evaluation

- Diarrhea controlled with reduced frequency and soft formed consistency
- Absence of fluid/electrolyte imbalance
- Compliance with dietary modifications
- Reduced use and/or reliance on laxatives
- Return to baseline bowel elimination pattern

Constipation, Fecal Impaction

Aging	Immobility	Lack of dietary	Laxative	Medications: iron,
Reduced activity		fiber/fluids	abuse	diuretics, calcium,
Decreased peristalsis				phosphate gels,
Weakness of				aluminum hydroxide,
abdominal muscles				Belladonna

↓   ↓   ↓   ↓   ↓

Infrequent passage of stool
Accumulation of feces in rectum

↓

Reabsorption of water from feces

↓

Hard, dry feces of small volume
Decreased bowel sounds, peristalsis
Straining at defecation
Feeling of rectal fullness

↓

Constipation

↓

Absence of bowel elimination over extended period of time

↓

Fecal impaction

Bowel Elimination Disorders

The elderly are often preoccupied with bowel elimination. Bowel motility, effects of medications and changes in the physiology of defecation contribute to the problems of constipation which may lead to fecal impaction or diarrhea which may lead to fecal incontinence. Important factors in the cause and treatment of these disorders include diet intake, fluid intake and activity/mobility. Autonomic nervous system control of intestinal motility may cause constipation while cortical inhibition may cause diarrhea. A bowel diversion is a procedure performed in association with resection in which a portion of the ileum (ileostomy) or colon (colostomy) is brought to the surface of the abdomen to create a diversion of fecal elimination. Ileal diversion include ileostomy, continent ileostomy, ileorectal anastomosis, and ileoanal reservoir. Colon diversion includes a single permanent ostomy.

MEDICAL CARE

Bulk laxatives: psyllium (Metamucil) PO to provide bulk to stool and promote peristalsis and bowel elimination

Stool softeners: docusate (Colace, Surfak) PO to soften and emulsify stool for easier removal

Suppositories: bisacodyl (Dulcolax), glycerin to irritate mucosa and stimulate peristalsis to promote elimination

Oil enema: Retention enema to soften impacted stool for easier removal

Antidiarrheals: diphenoxylate (Lomotil) PO to increase intestinal tone and decrease intestinal motility; kaolin and pectin (Kaopectate) PO to consolidate stool

Electrolyte replacements: potassium chloride (K-Lyte) PO to replace potassium loss in diarrhea

Abdominal x-ray: Reveals distention or obstruction of bowel

Proctosigmoidoscopy: Reveals rectal, sigmoid pathology

Barium enema: Reveals colon pathology

Stool examination: Reveals occult blood or culture revealing causative organism for diarrhea

Electrolyte panel: Reveals electrolyte imbalance especially potassium from fluid loss caused by diarrhea

NURSING CARE PLANS

Essential nursing diagnoses and plans associated with these conditions:

Risk for fluid volume deficit (151)

Related to: Excessive losses through normal or abnormal routes from diarrhea
Defining characteristics: I&O imbalance, frequent loose, watery stools, dry skin and mucous membranes, electrolyte imbalance, impaired thirst sensation

Risk for impaired skin integrity (246)

Related to: External factor of excretions, diarrhea
Defining characteristics: Reddened, irritated perianal skin, burning and soreness of perianal skin; redness, swelling, pain at peristonal site

Constipation (121)

Related to: Less than adequate dietary intake and bulk (soft diet)
Defining characteristics: Frequency less than usual pattern, hard-formed stool, decreased bowel sounds, less than usual amount of stool, palpable mass, reported feeling of rectal fullness, abdominal pressure, inability to chew and swallow foods containing bulk, cellulose

Related to: Less than adequate physical activity
Defining characteristics: Imposed bedrest, impaired physical mobility, immobility

Related to: Chronic use of medication and enemas
Defining characteristics: Use of laxatives, frequent bouts of constipation

Related to: Neuromuscular impairment from neurological disease
Defining characteristics: Decreased bowel sounds, impaired peristalsis, lack of awareness of defecation urge

Related to: Weak abdominal musculature
Defining characteristics: Unable to expel stool, straining at stool, incomplete stool elimination, general weakness and fatigue

Related to: Emotional status from neurological/psychological conditions
Defining characteristics: Confusion, agitation, cognitive deficit, lethargy, apathy, appetite impairment, depression

Related to: Musculoskeletal impairment from musculoskeletal disorders
Defining characteristics: Immobility, fracture with cast/traction, unable to use commode/toilet, activity intolerance, weakness, pain, discomfort

Diarrhea (122)

Related to: Dietary intake of soft, low residue diet
Defining characteristics: Increased frequency, increased bowel sounds, loose, liquid stools, fluid/electrolyte imbalance, cramping, urgency, fecal incontinence

Related to: Medications of laxatives, antibiotics
Defining characteristics: Frequent passage of stools, loose, liquid or watery stools, abdominal pain, cramping

Related to: Inflammation, irritation, or malabsorption of bowel from gastrointestinal disorders
Defining characteristics: Increased frequency of loose, liquid stools, cramping, increased bowel sounds, changes in color of stool, fever, malaise, blood, mucus, fatty substances in stool

SPECIFIC DIAGNOSES AND CARE PLANS

Colonic constipation

Related to: Less than adequate fluid, fiber intake and immobility (fecal impaction)
Defining characteristics: Abdominal distention, pain, lethargy, straining at stool, unable to pass stool, palpable mass by rectal examination, rectal pressure

Outcome Criteria

Complete removal of fecal impaction without trauma to rectal mucosa.

Interventions	Rationales
Assess for presence of fecal impaction by digital examination or abdominal palpation	Hard mass of stool palpated indicates impaction
Prepare to remove feces that is still soft and pliable by: • Placing client on left side in Sims position • Draping appropriately • Lubricating gloved fingers and insert into rectum	Removal of soft impaction promotes comfort and prepares for subsequent bowel movements

Interventions	Rationales
• Gently and carefully removing small amounts at a time with a circular rather than digging motion • Informing to take deep breaths during removal • Administering molasses or other carminitive enema after removing as much stool as possible • Informing to retain enema as long as possible to soften stool • Allowing to expel remaining stool with enema return	
Prepare to remove feces that is hard by: • Irrigating with 60 ml hydrogen peroxide or administer retention oil enema • Allowing to retain and when examination reveals that stool has softened, proceed with procedure to remove soft mass as outlined above	Necessary to break up feces or soften before removal to prevent damage to mucosa
Cleanse rectal area and proceed with bowel training regimen	Removal of impaction allows for bowel rehabilitation

Information, Instruction, Demonstration

Interventions	Rationales
Suggest rectal digital stimulation or glycerin suppository 30 minutes before scheduled defecation	Promotes defecation at specific time schedule to prevent recurrence of impaction

Interventions	Rationales
Inform to avoid enema, laxatives	Tends to compound the problem by causing constipation
Follow teaching for fluid, dietary and exercise inclusions	Promotes regular bowel elimination

Discharge or Maintenance Evaluation

• Absence of fecal impaction, bowel elimination pattern established
• Completed removal of fecal impaction

Bowel incontinence

Related to: Neuromuscular, musculoskeletal involvement (neurological disorder)
Defining characteristics: Involuntary passage of feces, decreased rectal sphincter tone

Related to: Depression, anxiety
Defining characteristics: Agitation, lethargy, apathy

Related to: Perception or cognitive impairment (neurological disorder)
Defining characteristics: Involuntary passage of feces, memory deficit, disorientation, fecal stains on clothing

Outcome Criteria

Control passage of stool.

Interventions	Rationales
Assess presence of diarrhea, fecal impaction, patency of rectal sphincter, awareness of urge to defecate, ability to control defecation	Provides data regarding presence or potential of bowel incontinence as aging causes change in muscle tone and reflex activity, sensory perception

Diarrhea, Bowel Incontinence

Stress	Malabsorption	Bacterial overgrowth (antibiotics)	Laxative abuse Irritated colon	Fecal impaction
				↓

↓   ↓   ↓   ↓   Fecal mass
in rectum

Increased water content of stool, increased motility of bowel

↓

↓

Large or small volume diarrhea   Absence of
defecation

↓

↓

Loose, watery, frequent stools   Relaxed sphincter
Abdominal cramping, flatulence   Dribbling of feces
Increased bowel sounds   from around
Tenesmus   impaction
Fluid/electrolyte imbalance   through anus
Weight loss

↓

Fecal incontinence
Soiling of clothing

Interventions	Rationales
Provide consistent elimination pattern before stool accumulates in rectum; remind to use bathroom or commode	Promotes emptying of bowel and prevents leakage of feces
Provide pads or waterproof garment if difficult to control fecal leakage; perianal pouch if appropriate	Protects clothing and prevents embarrassment
Change clothing immediately if soiled	Prevents embarrassment

Information, Instruction, Demonstration

Interventions	Rationales
Suggest sitting on commode or toilet 30 minutes after breakfast daily	Promotes bowel regularity and prevents bowel incontinence if feces removed from rectum
Inform of changes related to aging that result in bowel elimination problems	Promotes understanding and prevention of related problems
Avoid use of laxatives	May create urgency and incontinence of feces if unable to reach bathroom in time
Instruct in perineal exercises (Kegal)	Strengthens perineal muscles to increase tone

Discharge or Maintenance Evaluation

- Return of bowel control with absence of incontinence
- Compliance with bowel pattern regimen to reduce incontinence episodes

- Able to use commode, toilet before bowel incontinence occurs

Body image disturbance

Related to: Biophysical factors (colostomy/ileostomy, bowel incontinence)
Defining characteristics: Verbal response to actual change in structure and/or body function, negative feelings about colostomy/ileostomy and leakage of feces or intestinal drainage

Outcome Criteria

Improved body image with adaptation to presence of colostomy/ileostomy.

Interventions	Rationales
Assess for responses to colostomy or ileal diversion surgery, effect on lifestyle, coping behaviors	Provides information about effect on body image and ability to adapt to and manage changes in body function
Assess for feelings about altered bowel elimination and presence of stoma and appliance if used	Promotes open discussion about the change in bowel elimination pattern and special care requirements
Allow for expression of feelings about socializing and participation in care; ensure that bowel diversion will not interfere with usual activities or ADL	Promotes venting of feelings and participation in activities to prevent isolation, dependence on others for care

Information, Instruction, Demonstration

Interventions	Rationales
Suggest loose and fully styled clothing	Conceals ostomy appliance

Interventions	Rationales
Advise on methods to eliminate odor from colostomy/ileostomy drainage, use deodorizer if needed or tablets in the pouch	Prevents embarrassing odors
Avoid foods that are gas forming	Prevents cause of flatulence and odor from gas release

Discharge or Maintenance Evaluation

- Verbalization of improved body image and progressive adaptation to bowel diversion
- Uses clothing appropriate to change in body image
- Prevents embarrassment of odors

Knowledge deficit

Related to: Lack of information about care of colostomy/ilesotomy
Defining characteristics: Request for information about bowel diversion care

Outcome Criteria

Ability to perform appropriate care of colostomy/ileostomy.

Interventions	Rationales
Pathophysiology and bowel diversion anatomic changes, type of ostomy and consistency and characteristics of material eliminated	Provides information and rationale for functional pattern of bowel elimination
Dressing change and wound/stoma protection during bathing, use of skin barrier or sealant	Maintains clean dry wound and peristoma skin

Interventions	Rationales
Removal and application of appliance, pouch application and emptying with associated skin and stoma assessment and care (ileostomy and colostomy); include measurement of stoma for appliance fit	Ensures proper and safe care and use of ostomy supplies and skin protection/barriers to prevent leakage and skin breakdown
Colostomy irrigation daily or q2 days, setting-up equipment, solution and administration	Ensures bowel cleansing and trains for establishment of bowel elimination pattern
Instruct in draining and irrigating of continent ileostomy, clamping of catheter if in the stoma, insertion of catheter into stoma to drain reservoir into a toilet by gravity	Ensures correct method and schedule of emptying reservoir for ileal draining by catheter insertion to drain pouch as frequently as needed to prevent distention
Application of pad, catheter placement in reservoir at night, and connection to drainage device	Provides care of ileo-anal anastomosis post-operatively
Defecation prior to overdistention of rectum or to respond to urge to defecate to avoid incontinence while bowel adapts to change in pattern, include perianal cleansing and skin care	Ileorectal anastomosis and ileoanal reservoir bowel diversion procedures do not require stoma or appliance care as drainage is excreted via the colon
Proper cleansing of pouches/catheters, storage of reusable supplies	Minimizes odors from the ostomy and provides proper storage for subsequent use of supplies and equipment to care for various bowel diversions
Inform that stoma size will reach permanent status by 4 months	Prevents anxiety caused by changes in stoma

Interventions	Rationales
Cleanse peristomal or perianal skin with mild soap and warm water and gently pat dry after each exposure to fecal or other secretions	Promotes cleanliness and prevents irritation from intestinal secretions for those who only use a dressing over the stoma or if appliance worn
Referral to enterostomal therapist if needed	Provides problem-solving assistance to prevent complications
Suggest alternative sexual activities, covering stoma during sexual activity, possibility of sexual counseling	Assistive aids can enhance sexual satisfaction
Report any redness, swelling, or pain at stoma site, change in stoma and output characteristics, temperature elevation	Signs and symptoms of possible complications of bowel diversion

Discharge or Maintenance Evaluation

- Performs care of stoma, peristomal skin, irrigation, appliance removal and application
- Requests assistance and/or asks questions when needed
- Avoids dietary/fluid intake restrictions that can affect normal elimination via diversion
- Reports any signs and symptoms of infection, constipation, diarrhea

Cholecystitis, Cholelithiasis

Aging   Obesity   Dietary factors
                                                                               High fat intake

↓   ↓   ↓

Increased cholesterol into bile, storage of bile in gallbladder
Distention of gallbladder with excess bile

↓   ↓

Stasis of bile   Thickened and edematous gallbladder wall
↓   from exposure to concentrated bile
                                        Increased pressure and ischemia in gallbladder

Bile salts precipitation

↓   ↓

Cholelithiasis   Cholecystitis

↓   ↓

Gallstones in common bile duct (obstruction)   Fatty food intolerance
                                                       Nausea, vomiting, belching
                                                         Pain following eating
                                                              Indigestion

↓

Acute cholecystitis
↓

Biliary colic
Vomiting
Fever
Jaundice

Cholecystitis, Cholelithiasis

Gallbladder abnormalities are common in the aged because of problems in emptying bile. It contains a smaller volume of thicker, high cholesterol bile. The greatest risk to the elderly is obstruction of the cystic or common bile duct with stones causing jaundice, the decrease in absorption of fat-soluble vitamins, and a decrease in fat digestion.

MEDICAL CARE

Analgesics: meperidine (Demerol) IM, oxycodone (Percodan) PO for pain of inflamation

Anticholinergics: propantheline (Probanthine) PO to reduce spasms of gallbladder

Antiemetics: benzquinamide (Emete-Con) PO to reduce nausea and vomiting by depressing the chemoreceptor trigger zone

Hydrocholeretics: dehydrocholic acid (Decholin) PO to stimulate bile production and assist with fat and vitamin absorption

Vitamin supplements: vitamin A, D, E, K, to replace fat-soluble vitamins that are not absorbed in small intestine

Abdominal x-ray: Reveals calcified stones in gallbladder

Oral, IV cholangiography: Reveals patency of gallbladder and duct system and presence of stones

Ultrasonography: Reveals stones in gallbladder

CT scan: Reveals changes in bile ducts, presence of obstruction

Bilirubin: Reveals increases in direct and indirect measurements if obstruction present

Fecal urobilinogen: Reveals decreases in presence of obstruction as bilirubin is not present to convert to urobilinogen in intestine

NURSING CARE PLANS

Essential nursing diagnoses and plans associated with this condition:

Altered nutrition: less than body requirements (118)

Related to: Inability to ingest, digest or absorb nutrients because of biologic factors of obstruction of bile flow
Defining characteristics: Nausea, vomiting, bleeding tendency, anorexia, reduced food intake, steatorrhea, weight loss, abdominal pain or discomfort

Risk for impaired skin integrity (246)

Related to: Internal factor of altered pigmentation from common bile duct obstruction
Defining characteristics: Jaundice, pruritis, scratching

SPECIFIC DIAGNOSES AND CARE PLANS

Pain

Related to: Biological injuring agents (inflammation, obstruction, spasm)
Defining characteristics: Communication of pain descriptors, epigastric pain after eating in RUQ, heartburn, feeling of heaviness, intolerance to fatty foods, abdominal distention

Outcome Criteria

Pain eliminated or controlled.

Interventions	Rationales
Assess severity of pain, factors that precipitate pain	Provides information regarding chronicity of disease and partial or complete obstruction
Administer analgesic appropriate to severity of pain	Controls pain by interfering with CNS pathways
Position in low-Fowler's	Reduces pressure in upper abdomen
Note effect of anticholinergics	Relieves pain by relaxing smooth muscle and decreasing spasms of ducts
Provide quiet environment, backrub, relaxation techniques	Non-pharmacological measures to relieve pain

Information, Instruction, Demonstration

Interventions	Rationales
Inform to avoid fatty foods (butter, oils, cream, cheese, milk, fried foods)	Precipitates pain, nausea

Discharge or Maintenance Evaluation

- Absence of pain in RUQ
- Effective response from muscle relaxants and antispasmodics

Knowledge deficit

Related to: Lack of information regarding prevention of recurrence, symptoms to report

Defining characteristics: Request for information, verbalization of the problem and fear of repeat attacks

Outcome Criteria

Increased knowledge of preventive measures verbalized.

Interventions	Rationales
Assess for frequency of attacks, need for information and ability to perform actions independently	Provides basis for teaching and type of information needed
Inform to take vitamin supplement and bile salts if condition is chronic	Assists with digestion and fat-soluble vitamin replacement
Offer plan for weight reduction if overweight	Obesity is risk factor for chronic cholecystitis
Inform to refrain from scratching and add cornstarch to water for bathing; apply pressure to itchy areas instead of scratching	Prevents breaks in skin and allays itching
Assist to plan menus that eliminate fatty foods in diet	Fatty diet precipitates attack as fats are difficult to digest with reduced bile
Inform to report any easy bruising to skin or mucous membranes, yellow color to skin, sclera, dark urine, clay-colored stools	Lack of vitamin K absorption affects blood clotting; jaundice and clay-colored stools indicates obstruction as bile is reabsorbed or unable to reach intestines

Discharge or Maintenance Evaluation

- Absence of symptoms of obstruction
- Compliance with dietary regimen of reduced fats
- Appropriate reporting of signs and symptoms of recurrence of attack or obstruction

Diverticular Disease

Atrophy of the intestinal wall is an age related factor responsible for development of diverticular disease. It is a noninflamed outpouching of the mucosa of the large intestine and has a high incidence in the elderly population. Risk factors associated with the disease are age, obesity, hiatal hernia, stress, lack of dietary fiber and persistent constipation problems. Inflammation (diverticulitis) may complicate this condition when material becomes lodged in these pouches as a result of ingestion of rough, irritating foods, coughing, or straining at defecation.

MEDICAL CARE

Bulk laxatives: psyllium (Metamucil) PO to provide bulk to stool for easier movement through colon

Stool softeners: docusate (Surfak, Colace) PO to soften stool for easier passage and prevent constipation

Anticholinergics: propantheline (Probanthine) PO to control smooth muscle spasms of bowel

Anti-infectives: ampicillin (Amcil) PO or specific to identified organism if infection develops

Barium enema: Reveals pouches in bowel wall usually found in sigmoid section of colon

Stool specimen: Reveals occult blood and mucus present in bowel inflammation

NURSING CARE PLANS

Essential nursing diagnoses and plans associated with this condition:

Altered nutrition: less than body requirements (118)

Related to: Inability to digest food because of biologic factors from diverticular formation
Defining characteristics: Low residue dietary intake, material caught in pouches, inflammation of pouches in colon, weight loss, abdominal pain or cramping

Constipation (121)

Related to: Less than adequate intake of bulk from low residue intake
Defining characteristics: Hard formed stool, frequency less than usual pattern, decreased bowel sounds, palpable mass, flatulence

Diarrhea (122)

Related to: Dietary intake of soft, low residue diet and inflammation, irritation of bowel from rough, spicy foods
Defining characteristics: Loose liquid stools, increased frequency of stools, cramping, episodes alternating with constipation episodes

SPECIFIC DIAGNOSES AND CARE PLANS

Pain

Related to: Injuring biological agent (inflammation)
Defining characteristics: Communication of pain descriptors, pain in LLQ, abdominal guarding, tachycardia, hypotension, bradypnea

Outcome Criteria

Pain controlled or eliminated.

Colorectal Cancer

Aging   Familial polyposis   Lack of dietary fiber   History of ulcerative colitis
  ↓   ↓   ↓   ↓

Colon mass, unknown factor
↓

Uncontrolled cell growth
↓

Invasion of mucosal and submucosal layer
↓

Invasion of entire wall of colon
↓

Invasion of serosal layer with regional lymph node involvement

↓   ↓

Metastasis   Bleeding from bowel
↓   Palpated mass
                                     Change in bowel habits (constipation/diarhhea)
Liver   Bowel obstruction
Lungs   Pain (late symptom)
Bone
Lymphatic system

Diverticular Disease

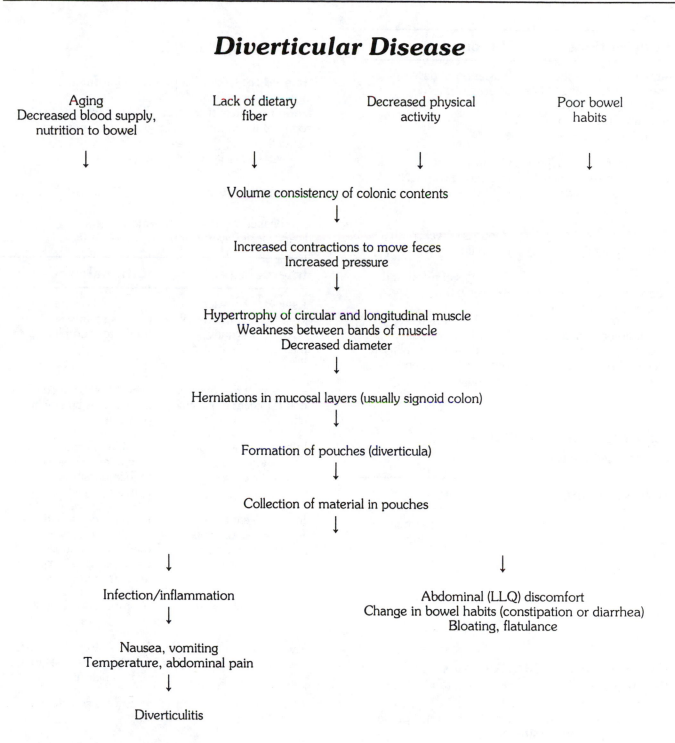

Aging
Decreased blood supply,
nutrition to bowel

Lack of dietary
fiber

Decreased physical
activity

Poor bowel
habits

↓ ↓ ↓ ↓

Volume consistency of colonic contents

↓

Increased contractions to move feces
Increased pressure

↓

Hypertrophy of circular and longitudinal muscle
Weakness between bands of muscle
Decreased diameter

↓

Herniations in mucosal layers (usually signoid colon)

↓

Formation of pouches (diverticula)

↓

Collection of material in pouches

↓

↓ ↓

Infection/inflammation

Abdominal (LLQ) discomfort
Change in bowel habits (constipation or diarrhea)
Bloating, flatulance

↓

Nausea, vomiting
Temperature, abdominal pain

↓

Diverticulitis

Interventions	Rationales
Assess for intermittent, cramping pain in LLQ or a steady, dull pain radiating to back, pain following meals	Indication of developing diverticulitis
Administer mild analgesic unless pain severe; avoid narcotic analgesic if possible	Controls pain by interfering with CNS pathways
Administer anticholinergics	Reduces bowel spasms and pain
Apply dry heat to abdomen; K-pad may be best choice	Promotes comfort and relieves pain
Maintain bedrest if pain becoming more severe; place on NPO status	Treatment for pain caused by diverticulitis to prevent nausea and vomiting

Information, Instruction, Demonstration

Interventions	Rationales
Inform to check effect of analgesics and antispasmolytics in controlling pain	Allows for adjustment of medication regimen
Relaxation techniques (music, imagery)	Provides distraction to relieve pain

Discharge or Maintenance Evaluation

- Absence of abdominal pain with appropriate analgesic administration

Knowledge deficit

Related to: Lack of exposure to information (potential for infection or diverticulitis)
Defining characteristics: Request for information, cognitive limitation, noncompliance of previous instruction

Outcome Criteria

Compliance with preventive measures for diverticulosis/diverticulitis.

Interventions	Rationales
Assess for knowledge of signs and symptoms of disease, preventive measures, treatment of disease	Provides basis for teaching plan and promotes compliance
Assess past episodes of bowel infection, lifestyle changes	Prevent recurrence of diverticulitis by teaching prevention
Inform of risk factors associated with disease and recurrence	Provide information to eliminate risk factors and reduce possibility of complications
Inform to eat high fiber foods and avoid nuts, food with seeds, raw fruits and vegetables	Prevents constipation and irritation to bowel mucosa, retention of small particles in pouches leading to infections
Maintain daily exercise program	Promotes bowel motility
Avoid stressful situations, use relaxation techniques	Reduce stress and anxiety which predisposes to diverticular disease
Maintain fluid intake of at least 2 L/day	Promotes soft stools
Formulate plan for bowel elimination program	Eliminates feces and prevents episode of diverticulitis

Interventions	Rationales
Instruct to report any bleeding from rectum, LLQ pain, flatulence, alternating diarrhea and constipation, elevated temperature	Indication of recurrence of diverticulitis

Discharge or Maintenance Evaluation

- Compliance with dietary, fluid and exercise program
- Absence of changes in bowel pattern
- Absence or relief of signs and symptoms of diverticular disease

Hiatal Hernia, Gastro-Esophageal Reflux

Shortening of   →   Congenital weakness   Obesity
esophageal sphincter   of hiatal muscle
         ↓   ↓   ↓

Incompetent lower   →   Increased intra-abdominal pressure
esophageal sphincter   ↓
         ↓

Backflow of gastric contents   Protrusion of stomach through opening in diaphragm
         ↓   ↓   ↓

Gastroesophageal reflux   Rolling hernia   Sliding hernia
         ↓   ↓

Decreased pH of esophagus   Assumes normal position
Denaturation of mucosa   of stomach in
         ↓   upright position
                                                               ↓

Inflammation of muscularis layer   Sudden position change
         ↓   Increased peristalsis
                                                          Overeating
Decreased esophageal clearance   Physical exertion
         ↓   ↓

Increased muscle damage   Heartburn
Increased reflux   Indigestion
         ↓   Regurgitation
                                                           Dysphagia
Esophagitis
         ↓

Indigestion
Heartburn
Regurgitation of sour/bitter material
Dysphagia
         ↓

Nocturnal reflux and aspiration
Permanent structure

Hiatal Hernia, Gastro-Esophageal Reflux

The aging esophagus decreases in motility and the synchronization and relaxation of its sphincters which delays the emptying of the esophagus of its contents into the stomach. The delay in emptying causes putrifaction of the food in the esophagus resulting in spasms and reflux. Hiatal hernia may cause or accompany gastric reflux. Both have a high incidence in the elderly population.

MEDICAL CARE

Antacids: aluminium hydroxide (Amphojel), magaldrate (Riopan) PO to neutralize gastric acid and increase lower esophageal sphincter tone

Cholinergics: metoclopramide (Reglan) PO to increase resting tone of esophageal sphrincter and tone and amplitude of upper gastrointestinal contractions which improves gastric emptying

H₂ blockers: cimetidine (Tagamet), ranitidine (Zantac) PO to reduce basal gastric acid secretion

Stool softeners: docusate (Colace) PO to soften stool and prevent increased intra-abdominal pressure by straining on defecation if constipated

Chest x-ray: Reveals hiatal hernia

Barium swallow: Reveals abnormalities in stomach, esophagus and diaphragm

Esophageal studies: Manometry reveals swallowing waves and recordings of lower esophageal pressure; pH recordings to reveal low, acidic results

NURSING CARE PLANS

Essential nursing diagnoses and plans associated with this condition:

Altered nutrition: less than body requirements (118)

Related to: Inability to ingest food because of biological factors of reflux
Defining characteristics: Heartburn, regurgitation, dysphagia, indigestion, inadequate intake, lack of interest or desire for food

SPECIFIC DIAGNOSES AND CARE PLANS

Anxiety

Related to: Change in health status (hernia and persistent reflux)
Defining characteristics: Communication of concerns regarding discomfort and need for accommodation in lifestyle changes, anxious, worried about complications

Outcome Criteria

Anxiety level reduced and maintained at acceptable level.

Interventions	Rationales
Assess level of anxiety associated with dietary changes, preventive measures needed to control reflux	Anxiety and depression common in aged and may become chronic if condition doesn't improve

Interventions	Rationales
Provide calm, supportive environment for expression of fears	Permits venting of feelings to relieve anxiety
Promote relaxation exercises and techniques	Reduces anxiety
Encourage to identify anxiety and methods to resolve feelings	Assists to cope and reduce anxiety

Information, Instruction, Demonstration

Interventions	Rationales
Inform of disease process and causes of symptoms	Knowledge promotes understanding and reduces anxiety

Discharge or Maintenance Evaluation

- Statements that anxiety is reduced
- Performs relaxation exercises when exposed to stress

Pain

Related to: Biological injuring agents (irritated esophageal mucosa and oral cavity from reflux)
Defining characteristics: Communication of pain descriptors, heartburn, dysphagia, regurgitation of acidic, putrified material

Outcome Criteria

Pain eliminated or controlled.

Interventions	Rationales
Assess oral tissue integrity, belching, heartburn, indigestion, pain over lower sternum	Persistent regurgitation causes irritation and burning to mucosa
Administer antacids, cholinergics	Neutralizes acidity of gastric reflux and increases tone of esophageal sphincter
Maintain upright position; elevate head of bed to semi-Fowler's for sleep	Sliding hernia remains in normal position if in upright position and gravity prevents reflux

Information, Instruction, Demonstration

Interventions	Rationales
Methods to prevent reflux by changing dietary regimen, correct administration of medications	Reflux is source of pain and discomfort
Rinse mouth after regurgitation	Removes irritating substances

Discharge or Maintenance Evaluation

- Reduced frequency of dyspepsia, heartburn, regurgitation
- Statements that oral and esophageal pain reduced

Knowledge deficit

Related to: Lack of information regarding reduction in reflux activity
Defining characteristics: Request for information, verbalization of the problem

Outcome Criteria

Increased knowledge of actions that reduce reflux.

Interventions	Rationales
Assess for information needed and ability to perform actions independently	Provides basis for teaching
Inform and assist with reduction in caloric intake	Overweight increases intra-abdominal pressure
Inform to eat small amounts of bland food followed by small amount of water and remain in sitting position 2-4 hours after meals; avoid eating last meal within 3-4 hours of bedtime	Less irritating and gravity assists in control of reflux
Inform that bending over, coughing, straining at defecation increases reflux of gastric content	Promotes comfort by decreasing intra-abdominal pressure which reduces reflux of gastric content
Inform to eat slowly and chew foods well; maintain high protein, low fat diet	Prevents reflux
Avoid hot and cold, spicy or gas-forming foods, citrus fruit	Increases acid production and that precipitates heartburn
Avoid alcohol, smoking, caffeine beverages	Increases acid production and may cause esophageal spasms
Inform to raise both arms fully extended toward ceiling before eating	Relieves spasms and allows for more comfort when eating
Inform to avoid tight fitting clothing around waist, heavy lifting, stooping or bending	Promotes comfort by reducing intra-abdominal pressure

Discharge or Maintenance Evaluation

- Statements of actions to take to prevent or reduce reflux
- Compliance with dietary inclusions and restrictions
- Increased knowledge of the importance of positioning during meals, sleep and work

Malnutrition

Stress Genetic factors Sedentary lifestyle	Anorexia Nausea	Impaired digestion Impaired malabsorption		Aging
↓	↓	↓	←	↓
Excessive caloric intake Decreased metabolic rate	Decreased caloric intake			Depression, isolation Dental, oral problems
↓	↓	→	↓	↓
Weight gain exceeding 20% of standard for age, height and frame			Nutritional deficiency ↓	
↓			Weight loss of 20% of baseline Anemia Vitamin deficiency Emaciation	
Overweight ↓				
Increase in body fat ↓				
Obesity				

Malnutrition

Age associated influences on nutrition may be physiological or psychological. They vary from abnormal mouth or dental factors, reduced metabolic rate, decreased energy, sensory and motor deficits, chronic diseases to isolation, depression, anxiety, grief, effect of medications and lack of interest and desire to eat. The result may be underweight (dietary deficiency) or overweight (caloric excess) which predispose the elderly client to potential injury, infection, bowel elimination problems, ineffective coping ability, fatigue, fluid/electrolyte imbalances, temperature variations, skin/mucous membrane impairment, body image/self-esteem deficits.

MEDICAL CARE

Multivitamins/Minerals: Replaces vitamin, mineral deficiencies if client is on restricted diet or nutritional intake lacks essential vitamins

Total protein and albumin: Reveals protein inadequacy

Fat and water soluble vitamins: Reveals decreased level of deficient vitamin(s)

Lipid panel: Reveals lipid, triglycerides, cholesterol level related to nutritional intake

NURSING CARE PLANS

Essential nursing diagnoses and plans associated with this condition:

Altered nutrition: less than body requirements (118)

Related to: Inability to ingest or digest food or absorb nutrients from biological or psychological factors

Defining characteristics: Body weight 20% or more under ideal for height and frame, inadequate intake, lack of interest or desire for food, depression, weakness, fatigue, isolation, oral disorder, dysphagia, chronic illness

Altered nutrition: more than body requirements (120)

Related to: Excessive intake in relationship to metabolic need of high caloric foods

Defining characteristics: Weight 10% over ideal for height and frame, sedentary activity level, decreased metabolic rate with increased food intake, eating in response to psychological stressors

Altered tissue perfusion: gastrointestinal (6)

Related to: Interruption of arterial flow from artherosclerosis

Defining characteristics: Reduced circulation and transport of nutrients needed to carry out digestion and absorption and transport from the intestines, weight loss

SPECIFIC DIAGNOSES AND CARE PLANS

Risk for infection

Related to: Malnutrition

Defining characteristics: Exposure to pathogens, inadequate nutrients reaching tissue to maintain integrity

Outcome Criteria

Absence of infection in pulmonary, renal, gastrointestinal or integumentary system.

Interventions	Rationales
Assess for temperature elevation, cough, yellow sputum, change in breathing pattern, urine that is cloudy and foul smelling, vomiting, diarrhea, redness, drainage from skin lesion or mucous membrane	Signs and symptoms of infection that result with nutritional and fluid deficiencies that fail to provide tissue and organs with protein, fats, carbohydrate, vitamins and minerals necessary for proper function of body's immune system and tissue building
Provide nutritional diet that fulfills daily requirements	Provides necessary nutrients to prevent infection
Provide rest and activities within limitations	Promotes health and assists to resist infection
Administer anti-infectives	May be prescribed to prevent or treat infection

Information, Instruction, Demonstration

Interventions	Rationales
Avoid exposure to URI or other infectious processes	Preventative measure to avoid upper respiratory infection
Proper handwashing before eating, after bathroom use	Removes transient flora from hands and prevents transmission of microorganisms

Discharge or Maintenance Evaluation

- Lungs clear on auscultation, sputum clear

- Urine yellow and clear, voided in appropriate amounts
- Absence of gastrointestinal discomfort, vomiting, diarrhea
- Skin intact without redness, irritation or lesions
- Mucous membranes pink, moist and intact

Body image disturbance

Related to: Biophysical factors (emaciated or obese appearance)
Defining characteristics: Verbal response to actual change in body structure, negative feelings about body, change in social involvement, depression

Outcome Criteria

Progressive return of positive body image.

Interventions	Rationales
Assess expression of feelings about appearance change, interest in appearance, negative statements about body, feelings of helplessness	Provides information regarding degree of anxiety and willingness to enhance appearance
Assess for coping and problem-solving skills and techniques that have worked in past	Provides postitve attributes to assist with increasing body image
Make appropriate adjustments in dietary intake, nutritional and caloric needs	Promotes needed weight gain or loss
Assist with makeup, hair care for women; shaving, hair shampoo for men	Enhances appearance
Suggest clothing that cover but do not accentuate appearance of thinness or obesity	Enhances appearance and body image acceptance
Assist to increase social interactions	Reduces isolation and sensory deprivation

Interventions	Rationales
Use praise, affection whenever possible	Increases feeling of self-worth and improves nurse-client relationship

Information, Instruction, Demonstration

Interventions	Rationales
Importance of dietary compliance	Method of returning to baseline weight to improve body image
Refer to counseling if anxiety or depression warrants treatment	Improves and supports psychological needs

Discharge or Maintenance Evaluation

- Statements that body image improved as weight problem corrected
- Statements of positive features of body appearance
- Statements of understanding of age-related changes that affect appearance and body image

Oral Disorders

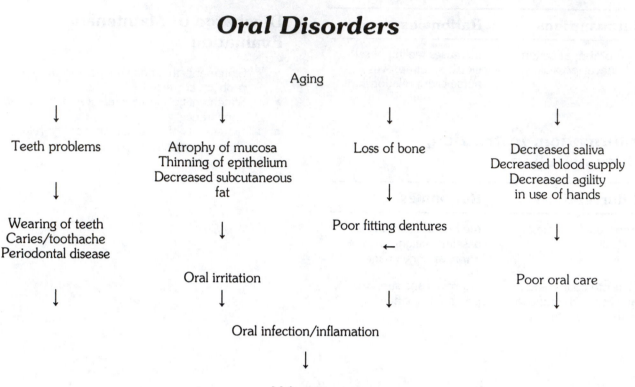

Aging

| Teeth problems | Atrophy of mucosa
Thinning of epithelium
Decreased subcutaneous
fat | Loss of bone | Decreased saliva
Decreased blood supply
Decreased agility
in use of hands |

Wearing of teeth
Caries/toothache
Periodontal disease

Poor fitting dentures

Oral irritation

Poor oral care

Oral infection/inflamation

Malnutrition
Halitosis
Xerostomia
Oral pain
Hyperemia
Tooth loss/dentures

Oral Disorders

Aging changes that affect oral structures and mucous membranes cause alterations in the gastrointestinal system as digestion begins with the mouth and teeth. Appetite and food ingestion is associated with tooth decay, wearing and loss, gum infection and loss of tooth support, dryness, varicosities and leukoplakia of the mucous membranes, loss of taste and smell perception and the progressive loss of calcium from the bone structure of the mouth. These contribute to the nutritional disorders found in the elderly population.

MEDICAL CARE

Anti-infectives: nystatin (Mycostatin) PO to treat fungal infections in mouth by interfering with cell wall synthesis

Dental x-ray: Reveals bone loss, caries in teeth

Oral culture: Reveals causative organism of mouth lesions, infection

NURSING CARE PLANS

Essential nursing diagnoses and plans associated with these conditions:

Altered nutrition: less than body requirements (118)

Related to: Ingestion and digestion of food
Defining characteristics: Anorexia, difficulty in chewing, poor fitting dentures, tooth loss or pain, sore, inflamed buccal cavity

Sensory/perceptual alterations: gustatory, olfactory (72)

Related to: Altered sensory reception, transmission and/or integration from neurological deficit, altered status of sense organs
Defining characteristics: Reported change in taste and smell acuity

SPECIFIC DIAGNOSES AND CARE PLANS

Altered oral mucous membrane

Related to: Mechanical trauma (ill-fitting dentures, nasogastric tube)
Defining characteristics: Oral lesions or ulcers, edema, hyperemia, oral pain or discomfort, thinning of epithelium of mucosa

Related to: Ineffective oral hygiene (inadequate strength to brush teeth and clean mouth)
Defining characteristics: Oral plaque, halitosis, carious teeth

Related to: Mouth breathing
Defining characteristics: Coated tongue, xerostomia, cracked lips

Related to: Infection (stomatitis, candida, periodontal disease)
Defining characteristics: Oral lesions or ulcers, leukoplakia, oral pain or discomfort, desquamation, gingivitis

Related to: Decreased salivation
Defining characteristics: Xerostomia, cracking oral mucosa and lips

Outcome Criteria

Oral mucous membrane intact and free of irritation and pain.

Interventions	Rationales
Assess teeth for pain, missing or loose teeth, fit of dentures and irritation caused by friction, fissures or cracks at corners of mouth, ability to chew	Osteoporosis, wearing of teeth from abrasion and erosion or grinding action associated with aging cause deterioration of structures that hold dentures in place; poorly fitting dentures may need relining periodically
Assess gums for redness, pain, bleeding with and without dentures	Indicates periodontal disease and potential for infection and tooth loss
Assess mucosa for lesions, dryness, pain, redness, bleeding, white coating, tongue for coating, size, involuntary movements, halitosis	Indicates poor oral hygiene and dryness from decreased saliva production or medication; mucosa, lips and tongue should be pink and moist
Provide oral care or assist with oral care daily and/or after meals	Promotes cleanliness and reduces odor
Remove plaque with soft brush and gentle flossing	Provides care if client unable to perform oral care
Remove secretions or mucus with saline solution or sodium bicarbonate solution; irrigate with hydrogen perioxide solution	Removes substances (mucin, damaged cells) if brushing not indicated or if stomatitis present
Clean dentures and soak in denture solution at night; remove all adhesive material	Cleans and freshens dentures to enhance appearance and prevent odor
Provide antiseptic mouthwash three times/day	Removes transient bacteria
Stimulate gums around remaining teeth	Promotes circulation to gums and prevents infection

Information, Instruction, Demonstration

Interventions	Rationales
Demonstrate and instruct in teeth brushing with soft brush, massaging of gums where teeth are missing, flossing and gum stimulation	Promotes clean oral cavity and prevents dental problems
Instruct in care of dentures before bedtime	Promotes cleanliness and preserves dentures
Inform of importance of dental visits and teeth repair	Preserves teeth and ensures proper fit of dentures
Inform of types of foods to eat if chewing is a problem and need for fluid intake of at least 2 L/day	Provides appropriate nutritional intake
Inform to remove dentures when eating or if mouth is painful in stomatitis	Prevents further irritation and pain to mucosa caused by chemotherapy
Inform to avoid smoking, hot liquids, alcohol in presence of stomatitis	Irritating to oral mucosa
Suggest artificial saliva	Provides relief from dry oral mucous membranes

Discharge or Maintenance Evaluation

- Oral mucosa pink, moist and intact
- Complies with daily oral and dental care as instructed
- Well-fitting dentures and/or teeth repair
- Ability to ingest and chew foods without pain or damage to mucosa or gums

Renal, Urinary, Reproductive System

Renal, Urinary, Reproductive Systems

Renal disease in the elderly occurs over a long period of time as a result of physiological conditions including renal disease, urinary tract infections, extrarenal diseases or trauma, organ atrophy, electrolyte and acid-base balance. Since the renal system has excretory, secretory and regulatory functions, it includes the process of urination and the changes that occur in aging that diminish this process. The most common effects found in the the older adult are incontinence, retention, impotence and urinary tract infection.

Included in this chapter is sexuality in the elderly. Although ageism attitudes about sexual expression is common in society, the need for love, intimacy and sex drive continue throughout senescence and remain an important and critical activity. The most common cause of a decline or cessation of sexual interest and activity is a change in the physical health of an individual and/or a partner.

An interrelationship exists among the three areas covered. The kidneys manufacture and excrete urine via the urinary tract. Problems of either the kidneys or in the organs of elimination may contribute to the dysfunction of either system. Disorders of the male or female reproductive tract commonly result in urinary problems of retention and incontinence as well as cause impotency.

GENERAL RENAL, URINARY, REPRODUCTIVE CHANGES ASSOCIATED WITH THE AGING PROCESS

Structural changes

Renal

- Decreased renal tissue growth causing a reduction in kidney size
- Decrease in number and increase in size of nephrons causing reduced renal function and efficiency
- Sclerosis of glomeruli and atrophy of afferent arterioles causing degeneration of glomeruli and glomerular filtration rate (GFR)
- Decreased cell mass causing decrease in intracellular body water; extracellular body water remains essentially the same
- Decreased water content of adipose tissue causing a decrease in total body water

Bladder

- Shape of bladder becomes more funnel shaped
- Decreased bladder capacity causing urinary frequency and nocturia
- Increased weakness of bladder and perineal muscles causing retention and stress incontinence in women
- Enlarged prostate in men causing frequency, urgency and dribbling of urine

Reproductive

- Decreased size of ovaries, uterus and cervix
- Decrease in subcutaneous fat causing a decrease in amount of and sagging breast tissue; flattening and folding of labia
- Muscle weakness causing uterine prolapse
- Shorter and narrower vagina; vaginal lining becomes atrophied, thinner and loses elasticity causing atrophic vaginitis, dyspareunia
- Increased size of prostate causing weaker contractions
- Decreased size and firmness of testes, thickening of testicular tubules causing decreased sperm production

Functional Changes

Renal

- Decreased renal blood flow, GFR and tubular function causing decreased ability to concentrate urine and clear body of drugs
- Decreased reabsorption of glucose and sodium conservation with acid-base abnormalities taking longer to return to normal levels
- Increased blood urea nitrogen (BUN) causing adjustments in evaluation of laboratory result norms in elderly
- Decreased muscle mass causing decreased creatinine production and creatinine clearance causing age adjustments in evaluating laboratory results

Bladder

- Decreased smooth muscle tone of bladder and sphincter relaxation causing frequency and nocturia
- Incomplete emptying of bladder causing urinary stasis and increased incidence of urinary tract infections
- Decreased inhibitory neural impulses to bladder causing decreased bladder contractions and voluntary control over bladder function resulting in incontinence

Reproductive

- Decreased estrogen secretion, follicular maturation and corpora lutea formation causing decreased stimulation to uterine lining
- As primary source of estrogen disappears, periodic dilatation of small blood vessels occurs causing "hot flashes"
- Decreased Bartholin gland secretion causing reduced mucus to lubricate vagina and dyspareunia
- Decreased testosterone secretion causing decreased sexual energy and viable spermatozoa
- Decreased volume and viscosity of seminal fluid causing decreased force of ejaculation
- Delay in achieving erection causing delayed orgasm and enhanced satisfaction for both sexes
- Sexual interest and activity are maintained in the elderly unless lack of privacy, illness or problems with sexual organs interfere with arousal, erection, ejaculation, vaginal lubrication or libido

ESSENTIAL NURSING DIAGNOSES AND CARE PLANS

Functional incontinence

Related to: Sensory, cognitive, or mobility deficits
Defining characteristics: Urge to void or bladder contractions strong enough to result in loss of urine before reaching commode, bathroom, lack of caretaker availability or interest, decreased bladder size and capacity, urgency, frequency, incontinent episodes, inability to find and reach commode, bathroom in time, lack of awareness, memory, comprehension, poor bladder control, unpredictable passage of urine

Outcome Criteria

Maintenance of continence as long as possible. Reduced number of incontinence episodes.

Interventions	Rationales
Assess physical and cognitive capabilities, voiding pattern (continent and incontinent), ability to sense that bladder is full and communicate desire to void, urgency or frequency, amount and time of day of fluid intake	Provides information about reasons for incontinence and establishes baselines as goal for continence
Assess for presence of chronic disease or procedures that may contribute to incontinence	Mental and physical disorders may prevent finding and using bathroom, walking to facility
Assess for medications such as diuretics, sedatives, psychotrophics	May reduce sensation to urinate or cause large amounts of urine to be excreted
Remind to use bathroom q2h and assist to sit or stand and to adjust clothing if necessary; keep call light within reach	Cognitive deficits causing forgetfulness is common and may need reminding to respond to urge for elimination
Provide privacy for urinary elimination; have bedpan, commode within easy access	Privacy is important to elderly clients and will promote continence
Schedule for toileting q2h during day and q4h during night at times identified in urinary pattern assessment	Promotes bladder training to prevent incontinence
Lengthen time periods for voiding as continence progresses	Allows client longer intervals between voidings
Promote fluid intake of at least 2 L/day (8-10 glasses)	Dilutes urine and prevents concentration of urine which is irritating to bladder
Reduce fluid intake 3 hours before bedtime; limit caffeine containing beverages	Prevents nocturia

Interventions	Rationales
Maintain consistency of schedule and approach, fluid intake spread over 24 hours	Promotes success of training program and prevents confusion
Provide pads or waterproof underwear; utilize aids such as condom catheter or female continence pouch	Protects clothing and prevents embarrassment of soiled clothes, serves as temporary measure to manage incontinence until bladder control regained
Insert indwelling catheter as a last resort	Incontinence that becomes impossible to control may require continuous drainage by indwelling catheter (total incontinence)

Information, Instruction, Demonstration

Interventions	Rationales
Instruct in Kegel exercises	Strengthens pelvic and perineal muscles to enhance control of urgency
Instruct in modification of environment with use of handrails, elevated toilet seat in bathroom; commode within easy assess	Promotes continence by adjustments that facilitate use of bathroom
Instruct and assist to plan toileting schedule and use of aids to control incontinence	Promotes independence and continence
Assist to follow a step by step method to find bathroom; place picture on door, alarm clock to remind to use bathroom	Serves to remind of bathroom location

Interventions	Rationales
Instruct in skin care with mild soap, warm water, drying well with soft cloth after each incontinence episode	Prevents skin irritation and breakdown

Discharge or Maintenance Evaluation

- Improved urinary continence with reduced incontinent episodes
- Use of toilet facilities, commode, bedpan with or without assistance
- Cooperation and compliance in training program
- Perineal skin intact and free of irritation
- Total continence achieved

Risk for fluid volume deficit

Related to: Extremes of age
Defining characteristics: Failure of regulatory mechanisms, weight gain or loss

Related to: Excessive losses through normal routes
Defining characteristics: Diarrhea, vomiting, output greater than intake, thirst, dry skin, mucous membranes, weakness, change in mental state

Related to: Loss of fluid through abnormal routes
Defining characteristics: Indwelling tubes, catheter, N/G tube

Related to: Deviations affecting access to, intake of, or absorption of fluids
Defining characteristics: Physical immobility, cognitive deficits, inattentive caretaker, weakness, altered intake

Related to: Factors influencing fluid needs
Defining characteristics: Hypermetabolic state, active loss

Related to: Medications
Defining characteristics: Diuretics, urinary frequency, increased fluid output greater than intake

Related to: Failure of regulatory mechanisms
Defining characteristics: Renal insufficiency, pituitary abnormality, increased urine output, dilute urine, sudden weight loss, increased Na, K levels

Outcome Criteria

I&O ratio within baseline determinations. Absence of dehydration and electrolyte imbalance.

Interventions	Rationales
Assess total fluid intake q4-8 h, and amount of and preferences in daily fluid intake (oral, parenteral), fluid restrictions	The elderly, in general, require at least 1750 ml fluids from liquids and food daily to maintain normal fluid balance and to carry out physiochemical body processes
Assess presence of diarrhea, vomiting, diaphoresis, tube aspirate, dehydration (thirst, hot, dry skin, lips and oral mucous membranes, poor skin turgor, oliguria, elevated temperature, weakness, sunken and mushiness of eyeballs)	The elderly are especially susceptible to fluid and electrolyte imbalance, acidosis, or alkalosis; these problems are caused by fluid losses
Assess urinary output q4-8 h, reduced Sp.gr. and concentrated appearance, color and odor	Output consists of sensible loss, blood loss, urine, stool, emesis, environmental factors
Assess medications taken and effect on intake and output	Diuretics increase fluid elimination and loss, sedatives may affect ability to obtain and take adequate fluids, urinary retention results from antihistamines, phenothiazines

Interventions	Rationales
Assess for weakness, paresthesias, leg cramps, muscle fatigue, pulse irregularity	Signs and symptoms of hypokalemia associated with K loss if not receiving a K-sparing diuretic (blocks secretion and loss of K in tubules)
Weigh daily or weekly as appropriate on same scale, time and wearing same clothing	Monitors for weight loss as a result of fluid loss
Provide at least 2 L/day fluids with inclusions of fruit juices and slushes, high-caloric beverages (increase intake over several days)	Replaces fluid loss and ensures adequate fluid intake and prevents fluid supplemental overload
Observe for confusion, sensory or cognitive deficits, mobility deficits, depression	Indicates ability to express thirst and/or obtain fluids
Monitor electrolytes, BUN, creatinine, protein, osmolality	Changes in blood and/or urine levels occur in presence of renal dysfunction affecting fluid output
Administer fluids via IV, N/G tube if appropriate	Replaces fluid loss if swallowing impaired or unable to retain fluids
Place fluids within reach and orient to placement; provide assistive aids for drinking	Provides fluids if forgetful or unable to obtain on own
Increase fluids if client resides in hot environmental temperatures and winds	Elderly have a reduced ability to adapt to temperature and fluid conservation which can result in rapid dehydration

Information, Instruction, Demonstration

Interventions	Rationales
Measuring I&O and kinds of foods to include in fluid intake (jello, custard, ice cream, soup/broth, liquid cereals, etc.)	Allows for ratio determination levels that may indicate changes in intake or medications
Weight weekly and reporting of abrupt changes	May indicate fluid deficit or excess
Amount of fluid daily and assist to schedule intake of 100-500 ml/hour or as appropriate for client, reducing intake before bedtime	Ensures intake over waking hours should be retained
Inform to avoid excessive salt intake in foods	May result in dehydration if fluid intake not adequate

Discharge or Maintenance Evaluation

- I&O maintained at levels based on individually determined baselines
- Baseline weight maintained
- Electrolytes within normal levels, especially potassium
- Absence of dehydration with fluid intake appropriate to losses
- Urinary output yellow in color, clear, at least 30 ml/hour
- Adequate amounts of fluids available and accessible for intake

Chronic Renal Failure

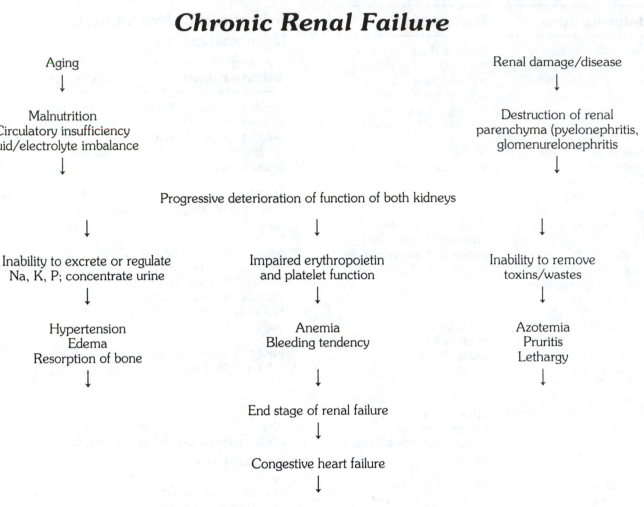

Aging
↓

Malnutrition
Circulatory insufficiency
Fluid/electrolyte imbalance
↓

Renal damage/disease
↓

Destruction of renal
parenchyma (pyelonephritis,
glomenurelonephritis
↓

Progressive deterioration of function of both kidneys

↓

↓

↓

Inability to excrete or regulate
Na, K, P; concentrate urine
↓

Impaired erythropoietin
and platelet function
↓

Inability to remove
toxins/wastes
↓

Hypertension
Edema
Resorption of bone
↓

Anemia
Bleeding tendency

↓

Azotemia
Pruritis
Lethargy
↓

End stage of renal failure
↓

Congestive heart failure
↓

Oliguria or anuria
Osteomalacia/osteoporosis/fractures
Asterixis
Encephalopathy/coma
Skin breakdown/uremic frost
Gastrointestinal bleeding
Metablic acidosis
Pericarditis
Dyspnea, Kussmall's respirations

Chronic Renal Failure

Chronic renal failure is the progressive reduction in the excretory function of both kidneys. Prognosis in the elderly depends upon the cause of the failure; poor if kidney parenchyma is involved and better if obstruction or a reversible disease is present. Overall, in the elderly, circulatory problems, dehydration, malnutrition, anemia, fluid and electrolyte problems, infection and fever contribute to the renal impairment that finally leads to accumulation of uremic toxins that affect the function of all organs.

MEDICAL CARE

Vitamins: Multivitamin preparation to supplement restrictive diet

Antipruritics: diphenhydramine/pseudoephedrine (Benadryl) PO to relieve itching

Diuretics: hydrochlorothiazide (Hydro-Diuril), furosemide (Lasix) PO to relieve edema and assist in excretion of Na, Cl, K, water by action on the renal tubular epithelium

Iron: iron sulfate (Feosol), folic acid (Folvite) PO to treat anemia

Calcium: calcitriol (Rocaltrol), calcium gluconate as replacement to treat hypocalcemia; given with vitamin D

Antacids: aluminum hydroxide (Amphojel), calcium carbonate (Titralac) PO to bind to dietary phosphates

Cation exchange resin: sodium polystyrene sulfonate (Kayexalate) PO in 20% sorbitol solution or as retention enema in 10-20% glucose solution to bind to K

X-ray: Kidney, ureters, bladder (KUB) revealing size, shape, placement of organs

Intravenous pyelogram, retrograde pyelogram: Reveals degree of renal function

Renal CT scan: Reveals kidney blood flow, glomerular and tubular function

Ultrasound: Reveals obstruction or masses

Electrolyte panel: Reveals increased K, Na, P and decreases in Ca, BUN

Renal function studies: BUN, uric acid, creatinine. Reveals increases as renal failure progresses

CBC: Hct, Hgb, RBC decreases as result of anemia

Urinalysis: Reveals fixed specific gravity, proteinuria, glycosuria, fixed osmolality

Creatinine clearance: Reveals a decrease as renal function decreases

NURSING CARE PLANS

Essential nursing diagnoses and plans associated with this condition:

Fluid volume excess (8)

Related to: Compromised regulatory mechanism from renal insufficiency
Defining characteristics: Edema, weight gain, oliguria or anuria, azoturia, blood pressure changes, sodium retention

Altered nutrition: less than body requirements (118)

Related to: Inability to ingest foods from dietary protein restriction
Defining characteristics: Anorexia, nausea, vomiting, accumulated nitrogen wastes

Risk for impaired skin integrity (246)

Related to: External factors of immobility and excretion of urea, internal factor of alteration in nutritional status from malnutrition
Defining characteristics: Pruritis and scratching, uremic frost on skin, dry skin, pressure on susceptible areas, emaciation, pale, sallow color

Altered thought processes (70)

Related to: Physiological changes from electrolyte imbalance, uremic encephalopathy
Defining characteristics: Lethargy, memory deficit, asterixis, delirium, seizures, coma

Sexual dysfunction (181)

Related to: Altered body function from renal failure
Defining characteristics: Impotence and loss of libido in males, amenorrhea and loss of libido in females

Constipation (121)

Related to: Less than adequate intake from fluid restrictions, less than adequate physical activity from weakness
Defining characteristics: Hard-formed stool, less frequent bowel elimination, abdominal or rectal fullness, decreased bowel sounds

SPECIFIC DIAGNOSES AND CARE PLANS

Ineffective individual coping

Related to: Multiple life changes (loss of independence, limitations on lifestyle, chronic disease)

Defining characteristics: Inability to meet basic needs, dependency, chronic fatigue, worry, anxiety, poor self-esteem, verbalization of inability to cope

Outcome Criteria

Anxiety, worry, fatigue reduced; increased independence in activities and decision-making process.

Interventions	Rationales
Assess coping methods, use of defense mechanisms, feelings about lifestyle changes, any losses associated with illness, ability to ask for help	Allows for interventions that promote control over life and ability to cope with long-term illness
Assist to identify positive defense mechanisms and promote their use; new behaviors to be learned	Use of defense mechanisms that have worked in the past increases ability to cope and promotes self-esteem
Provide environment that allows for free expression of concerns and fears	Encourages trust and relieves anxiety and worry
Assist to set short- and long-term goals; provide positive feedback regarding progress and focus on abilities rather than disabilities	Promotes self-worth and responsibility

Information, Instruction, Demonstration

Interventions	Rationales
Inform that compliance with treatment regimen reduces complications/progression of disease	Maintains health status

Interventions	Rationales
Refer to support group or counseling if appropriate; involve family members if client desires	Provides information and support from others with similar experiences
Relaxation techniques	Reduces stress and anxiety
Problem-solving approaches and techniques; new ways or methods to adapt to chronic illness	Promotes coping ability with lifestyle changes

Discharge or Maintenance Evaluation

- Uses appropriate coping mechanisms and problem solving methods in adapting to functional losses
- Asks for assistance when needed
- Seeks level of independence appropriate with activity tolerance and coping ability
- Statements that anxiety, worry, decreasing and feels more in control and capable of making decisions regarding health status and functional limitations

Activity intolerance

Related to: Generalized weakness (aging process, fatigue, chronic illness)
Defining characteristics: Communication of fatigue or weakness, presence of anemia, uremia, inability to maintain usual routines (ADL)

Outcome Criteria

Performance of activities at optimal level within limits set for independent ADL activity.

Interventions	Rationales
Assess tolerance for activity, expression of fatigue	Promotes activities without compromising physiological functions of involved systems
Assess response to existing or new activity; assist to identify tolerable level of activity without fatigue	Maintains baselines for activity tolerance while promoting participation in ADL independently
Maintain bedrest during symptomatic periods; progressively increase activity tolerance by independent movement in bed, active ROM, sitting up in bed, in chair, ambulating to bathroom with daily increases in distance	Promotes increasing activity without excessive energy expenditure
Assist with ADL activities based on expression of fatigue; allow to progress gradually, daily and incorporate ROM	Conserves energy while increasing or preserving endurance
Plan for rest periods during day without interruptions	Rest required to prevent depletion of energy

Information, Instruction, Demonstration

Interventions	Rationales
Plan time to perform activity by resting after each step, i.e., wash face, rest, brush teeth, rest	Conserves energy and prevents fatigue by pacing activities
Suggest exercises that are comfortable and within ability and preference	Promotes compliance and satisfaction associated with success

Discharge or Maintenance Evaluation

- Performs daily walking, rests when fatigued
- Increases ADL within scheduled limits
- Statements that energy level and endurance increased
- Schedules rest periods during day for 30 minutes-1 hour 2-3 times/day

Ineffective family coping: compromised

Related to: Prolonged disease or disability progression that exhausts supportive capacity of significant people (progressive dependence of client)
Defining characteristics: Fatigue, chronic anxiety, stress, social isolation, financial insecurity, expression of inadequate understanding of crisis and client's responses to health problem and necessary supportive behaviors

Outcome Criteria

Increased coping ability as client's care needs increase.

Interventions	Rationales
Assess knowledge of disease and erratic behaviors, possible physical/ emotional needs and reactions of client	Knowledge will enhance the family's understanding of the care associated with the disease and development of coping skills and strategies
Assess for level of fatigue, reduced social exposure of family, feelings about role reversal in caring for parent and increasing demands of client	Long-term needs of client may affect physical and psychosocial health of caregiver, economic status and prevent family from achieving own goals in life
Provide for opportunity of family to express concerns and lack of control of situation	Promotes venting of feelings and reduces anxiety

Interventions	Rationales
Assist in defining problem and use of techniques to cope and solve problems	Provides support for problem-solving and management of own fatigue and chronic stress
Assist to identify client's reactions and behaviors and reasons for them	May indicate need for anticipatory care and allow for interventions to prevent or reduce frustration

Information, Instruction, Demonstration

Interventions	Rationales
Demonstrate techniques to assist client with self-care needs of personal hygiene, dressing, eating and toileting	Assist family to provide personal care while conserving their energy
Demonstrate use of aids for walking, protecting the skin, eating, sleeping, remove environmental hazards	Assists family to prevent injury to client
Inform of need to maintain own health, social contacts	Fatigue, isolation, anxiety will affect the physical health and care capabilities of the caregiver
Suggest social worker referral if appropriate	Provides assistance for economic problems and respite services; need for long-term care facility

Discharge or Maintenance Evaluation

- Optimal health of family members, caregiver
- Statements of satisfactory contact with support group and/or professionals
- Statements that knowledge about disease and care of client increased and feeling more in control of situation

- Statements that anxiety reduced and coping and problem-solving techniques, relaxation techniques utilized
- Participating in diversional activities and maintaining social contacts

Risk for injury

Related to: Internal biochemical factor of regulatory function (electrolyte imbalance)
Defining characteristics: Increased Na, K, Cl, PO_4 levels, decreased Ca levels, fluid retention

Related to: Abnormal blood profile (decreased Hb, thrombocytopenia, leukopenia
Defining characteristics: Elevated temperature, infection, immunosuppression, inability of kidneys to excrete K, Na, resorption of Ca by bone, anemia

Outcome Criteria

Electrolyte imbalances corrected and maintained. Absence of respiratory, urinary infection, bleeding tendency.

Interventions	Rationales
Assess weakness, flaccidity of muscles, abdominal cramping with diarrhea, irregular pulse	Indicates hyperkalemia as renal tubular function decreases; electrolyte balance more easily disturbed and imbalances are more difficult to reverse in the elderly and Na, K and Cl are major influences in maintaining electrolyte balance
Assess for lethargy, weakness, restlessness, increased tendon reflexes	Indicates hypernatremia as nephrons lose ability to filter Na
Assess muscle cramping, numbness in fingers and toes, mentation changes	Indicates hypocalcemia as kidneys unable to metabolize vitamin D needed for Ca absorption and resorption of Ca by bones

Interventions	Rationales
Assess muscle cramping, paresthesia	Indicates hyperphosphatemia as kidneys unable to excrete PO_4
Assess for hematemesis, ecchymosis, prolonged bleeding from mucous membranes, injections	Altered platelet function and coagulation levels result in bleeding tendencies especially of gastrointestinal tract, skin
Monitor RBC, Hct, Hb for decreases	Anemia is a result of decreased erythropoietin by the kidneys affecting production of RBC by bone marrow; nutritional deficiencies also contribute to anemia (iron)
Restrict Na and K intake to 500-2000 mg/day and 1000-1500 mg/day respectively	Reduced renal function results in Na and K retention causing need to decrease daily intake
Avoid invasive procedures if possible	Prevents introduction of microorganisms and trauma causing prolonged bleeding
Perform handwashing and sterile technique for all procedures	Prevents infections in immunosuppressed condition
Provide oral care with soft brush, gentle brushing and mouthwash, use of electric razor	Prevents trauma to skin and mucous membranes that cause bleeding
Cleanse perineal area after each elimination, wipe from front to back in female	Prevents infection caused by bowel excreta contamination

Information, Instruction, Demonstration

Interventions	Rationales
Avoid contact with those with infections	Reduces infection potential
Avoid blowing nose hard, straining at defecation; avoid aspirin	Increases potential for bleeding
Use electric razor, soft tooth brush or soft applicator to clean teeth and gums	Reduces potential for break in skin and bleeding
Maintain clear pathways, avoid rushing, use rails and other aids during activities	Reduces possibility of falls
Avoid foods including table salt, snack foods, bacon, prepared meats, MSG in foods; bananas, tomatoes, fruit juices, potatoes; peas, corn, poultry	Foods high in Na, PO_4 and K should be restricted
Include dairy foods in diet	Foods high in Ca should be encouraged to replace deficiency
Report any change in breathing, sputum color; cloudy, foul smelling urine	Indicates respiratory or urinary infection

Discharge or Maintenance Evaluation

- Verbalizes precautions to take to prevent infection, bleeding or trauma from falls
- Plans menu of low Na, K, PO_4 and high Ca diet with statements of what foods to include and avoid
- Absence of excessive blood loss, infection
- Absence of symptoms of electrolyte imbalance
- Reports changes in mentation, symptoms of infection

Knowledge deficit

Related to: Lack of exposure to information (renal dialysis)
Defining characteristics: Verbalization of the problem, request for information

Outcome Criteria

Appropriate knowledge of dialysis procedure to clear body of metabolic wastes.

Interventions	Rationales
Assess knowledge of disease, reason for and procedure for dialysis prescribed (peritoneal or hemodialysis)	Provides information for teaching plan without repetition to promote understanding and compliance of medical regimen
Provide explanations and information in clear and simple language that is understandable; provide limited amounts of information over periods of time rather than large amounts at one sitting	Reduces potential for noncompliance of medical regimen related to cognitive ability to understand
Include caregiver/family in all teaching	Promotes understanding of family so support can be provided
Allow exposure to supplies and equipment used in dialysis	Promotes understanding of procedure to allay anxiety and fear of unknown
Inform of importance of adhering to having laboratory tests, keeping appointments with physician and dialysis schedule; benefits provided by government for those receiving dialysis	Promotes understanding and compliance to prolong state of wellness; dialysis may be performed 3 times/week and is prescribed when condition cannot be managed by conservative treatment

Discharge or Maintenance Evaluation

- Verbalizes knowledge and understanding of dialysis procedure
- States importance of maintaining dialysis schedule
- Adheres to physician and laboratory appointments as scheduled
- Receives government subsidy for dialysis therapy

Menopause

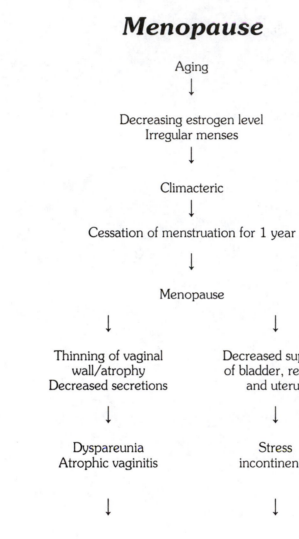

Aging
↓

Decreasing estrogen level
Irregular menses
↓

Climacteric
↓

Cessation of menstruation for 1 year
↓

Menopause

↓   ↓   ↓   ↓

Vasodilation   Thinning of vaginal   Decreased support   Alkaline vaginal
     ↓   wall/atrophy   of bladder, rectum   secretions
                  Decreased secretions   and uterus

Hot flahses   ↓   ↓   ↓

     ↓   Dyspareunia   Stress   Vaginal infection
                   Atrophic vaginitis   incontinence

Insomnia   ↓   ↓   ↓
     ↓

                          Nervousness
                          Depression
                          Osteoporosis

Menopause

Menopause is the cessation of menses resulting in reproductive senescence. The period leading up to this irreversible event is called the climacteric and is characterized by the decline of estrogen production by the ovaries until there is not enough to cause the endometrium to grow and shed. It is believed that at menopause, estrogen is secreted by nonovaraian sources (adrenal glands).

MEDICAL CARE

Estrogen: conjugated estrogen (Premarin) PO as replacement therapy to relieve symptoms and prevent osteoporosis

Vaginal smear: Reveals atrophy and lack of superficial cells

NURSING CARE PLANS

Essential nursing diagnoses and plans associated with this condition:

Sleep pattern disturbance (77)

Related to: Internal factors of psychological stress from menopause
Defining characteristics: Hot flashes, interrupted sleep, anxiety, depression, emotional lability, decreased REM sleep, nervousness

Sexual dysfunction (181)

Related to: Altered body structure and function from decreased estrogen secretion
Defining characteristics: Thin, dry vaginal mucosa, dyspareunia, slight bleeding during sexual intercourse, verbalization of problem, avoidance of engaging in sexual intercourse

SPECIFIC DIAGNOSES AND CARE PLANS

Stress incontinence

Related to: Degenerative changes in pelvic muscles and structural supports associated with increased age (aging)
Defining characteristics: Urinary urgency, urinary frequency, reported dribbling with increased abdominal pressure (cough, sneezing)

Outcome Criteria

Absence of accidental loss of urine.

Interventions	Rationales
Assess for incontinence associated with coughing, laughing, sneezing, lifting objects	Increased intra-abdominal pressure causes involuntary loss of urine when pelvic support organs are weakened by aging, catheter use or vaginal childbirth
Provide pads or waterproof underwear as appropriate	Prevents wetting of clothing and embarrassment

Information, Instruction, Demonstration

Interventions	Rationales
Inform of reason for dribbling, incontinence	Provides understanding of the problem for intervention and prevention planning

Interventions	Rationales
Instruct in perineal muscle strengthening (Kegel exercises) to be performed for 10 minutes QID or plan realistic schedule to follow	Improves muscle and sphincter tone and control over urine loss
Inform that contracting perineal muscles before coughing or sneezing may decrease or eliminate incontinence	Prevents increased intra-abdominal pressure which leads to urine loss

Discharge or Maintenance Evaluation

- Absence or progressively reduced incontinence
- Practices exercises according to planned instruction
- Ability to prevent incontinence episode associated with coughing, sneezing or laughing

Risk for infection

Related to: Inadequate primary defenses (traumatized tissue, change in pH secretions)
Defining characteristics: Change to alkaline secretions in vagina, decreased estrogen levels secreted, thinning of vaginal mucosa, atrophy of vaginal mucosa

Outcome Criteria

Absence of vaginal discomfort or infection.

Interventions	Rationales
Assess vagina and genitalia for itching, burning, pain, lack of secretions (dryness) or foul smelling secretions	Changes associated with aging predispose to easily traumatized and susceptibility to infection of vaginal mucosa (atrophic vaginitis)

Interventions	Rationales
Administer estrogen cream by vaginal applicator or suppository	Provides estrogen replacement and moisture to vagina to treat atrophic vaginitis
Secure vaginal smear for culture; administer anti-infective if culture positive via vaginal suppository	Identifies infectious organism if present

Information, Instruction, Demonstration

Interventions	Rationales
Instruct to apply water soluble lubricant to genitalia and vagina	Treats dryness
Instruct to avoid tight girdles or other tight clothing; wear cotton underwear	Irritates genitalia, cotton more porous and prevents dampness
Instruct to cleanse frequently, wash genitalia from front to back	Promotes comfort and prevents introduction of microorganisms
Inform to avoid use of douches, sprays, irritating soaps	Prevents alteration in pH of vagina and irritation of genitalia
Recommend yearly gynecological checks and Pap smear	Identifies presence of cancer and ensures gynecological health

Discharge or Maintenance Evaluation

- Correct administration of estrogen therapy, oral or vaginal
- Verbalizes increased comfort and absence of symptoms of infection
- Practices proper health practices in genitalia and vaginal care
- Absence of vaginal infection or trauma

Self-esteem disturbance

Related to: Biophysical factors (loss of reproductive capability, hormonal changes)
Defining characteristics: Self-negating verbalizations, loss of self-worth, expressions of guilt, depression, boredom, anxiety, insomnia, hot flashes, nervousness, change in self-perception of role

Outcome Criteria

Expresses feeling of reduced frustration, anxiety, nervousness and enhanced feeling of self-worth during adjustment to menopause.

Interventions	Rationales
Assess expressions of negative feelings, uselessness, self-worth, chronic anxiety or depression, general complaints about present status in life	Menopause creates more difficulty for women who feel that child-bearing is main reason for existence and self-worth, loss of reproductive ability then results in deeper emotional consequences
Encourage expression of feelings in nonjudgmental environment	Provides venting of concerns and reduces anxiety; trusting relationship with client

Information, Instruction, Demonstration

Interventions	Rationales
Inform that feelings and symptoms caused by decrease in hormone secretion are not unusual	Promotes understanding of problem for resolution and/or acceptance
Suggest referral to counseling for chronic anxiety or depression if not improving	Prevents prolonged depression and permanent emotional disability

Discharge or Maintenance Evaluation

- Expresses improved self-esteem and self-worth
- Reduced anxiety and nervousness
- Increased comfort as hot flashes controlled and sleep pattern returned
- Verbalizes adjustment to climacteric and subsequent menopause changes

Prostatic Hyperplasia

Aging

↓

Sexual hormone imbalance
Enlargement of prostate
Nodules in periurethral region

↓

Compression of urethra

↓

Partial or complete obstruction of urine flow

↓

Decreased stream
Difficulty in voiding
Urinary retention and overdistention
Frequency, nocturia
Overflow incontinence

↓

Destructive changes in bladder wall

↓

Herniation/diverticula of bladder wall

↓

Stasis of urine

↓

Urinary tract infection
Hydronephrosis

Prostatic Hyperplasia

A common problem of the aging male is prostatic hypertrophy or hyperplasia. It is the benign condition of an enlarged prostate gland leading to varied symptoms associated with urination which, if unchecked, finally may cause partial or complete urinary obstruction and chronic urinary bladder infections. The usual onset occurs between the ages of 60 and 70 and, as with any problem of the reproductive system, is a great source of anxiety for most men.

MEDICAL CARE

Anti-infectives: amoxicillin (Amoxil), ampicillin (Amcill), sulfisoxazole (Gantrisin) PO for associated urinary bladder infection if present

Rectal examination: Reveals enlarged prostate gland

Cytoscopy: Reveals amount of enlargement and obstruction by prostate and presence of small areas of hemorrhage

Intravenous pyelogram: Reveals prostate enlargement and effect on renal function if obstruction present

Urodynamic tests: Reveals urethral obstruction to urine flow

Urinalysis, routine and culture: Reveals hematuria, infectious agents and identifies them for treatment

Blood urea nitrogen (BUN): Reveals increases if hypertrophy is longstanding or if hydronephrosis is present

Prostatectomy: Surgical removal of all or part of the prostate gland by transurethral (most common), suprapubic or retropubic resection

NURSING CARE PLANS

Essential nursing diagnoses and plans associated with this condition:

Sleep pattern disturbance (77)

Related to: Internal factors of enlarged prostate gland
Defining characteristics: Interrupted sleep, anxiety, nocturia

Sexual dysfunction (181)

Related to: Biopsychosocial alteration of sexuality from altered body structure or function of obstructed urethra, prostatectomy
Defining characteristics: Verbalization of the problem, actual or perceived limitation imposed by disease, anxiety

SPECIFIC DIAGNOSES AND CARE PLANS

Urinary retention

Related to: Obstruction to urinary flow (enlarged prostate compressing on urethra)
Defining characteristics: Bladder distention, small, frequent voiding, dribbling, residual urine, overflow incontinence, nocturia, urgency, sensation of bladder fullness

Outcome Criteria

Return to or maintenance of urinary flow.

Interventions	Rationales
Assess I&O ratio, urinary frequency, urgency, dribbling and bladder distention by palpation	Incomplete voluntary control over bladder function and decreased bladder capacity causes frequency and nocturia which is further compromised when an enlarged prostate compresses against the urethra
Prepare for catheterization or catheterize if unable to void or after voiding to check for residual urine	May need a retention catheter inserted by physician or nurse (policy dependent) if unable to void if obstruction present; may be done to determine residual urine as result of partial obstruction and retention
Offer fluids of at least 2 L/day (8-10 glasses); decrease intake in evening and before sleep	Prevents dehydration and urinary bladder infection

Information, Instruction, Demonstration

Interventions	Rationales
Inform to void as soon as the urge is felt	Reduces urinary stasis and retention
Avoid caffeine and alcohol beverages	Increases prostatic symptoms
Instruct to see physician for periodic checks to evaluate prostate and symptoms if present	Provides early detection and treatment for prostatic conditions
Instruct to drink fluids daily of up to 2 L/day regardless of symptoms	Reducing fluid intake does not reduce symptoms and predisposes to infection

Interventions	Rationales
When away from home, be aware of location of bathroom, void before leaving home	Provides immediate voiding when needed and prevents embarrassment of dribbling and wetting clothing

Discharge or Maintenance Evaluation

- Decreased urgency, frequency, nocturia
- Complete or improvement in emptying of bladder
- I&O ratio within baseline determinations
- Urinary flow established

Risk for infection

Related to: Inadequate primary defenses (stasis of body fluids, invasive procedure (indwelling catheter)
Defining characteristics: Elevated temperature, cloudy urine, foul smelling urine, positive urine culture, frequency, dysuria, burning

Outcome Criteria

Absence of urinary bladder infection.

Interventions	Rationales
Assess presence of urinary retention, residual urine	Urinary stasis predisposes to infection
Assess presence of indwelling catheter, cloudy and foul smelling urine in urine container of closed system	Early detention of urinary bladder infection allows for immediate treatment before infection spreads to kidney (pyelonephritis)
Obtain clean catch urine specimen or remove from catheter for culture	Identifies infectious agent or evaluates effect of anti-infective therapy

Interventions	Rationales
Maintain proper catheter care: • Avoid kinking of catheter, lying on catheter to ensure patency • Empty container when two-thirds full • Maintain tubing and container below insertion level • Perform cleansing and catheter care at meatal site • Handle catheter gently	Prevents stasis, backflow of urine that causes infection
Perform handwashing before giving catheter care	Prevents transmission of bacteria at entry site
Change catheter according to policy or when needed using aseptic technique	Prevents infection from contamination by catheter insertion

Information, Instruction, Demonstration

Interventions	Rationales
Instruct in proper handwashing	Removes bacteria from hands and prevents transmission of bacteria
Advise to report frequency, dysuria, burning on urination, change in urine characteristics	Permits treatment of urinary Infections
Advise to report difficulty in urinating, frequency of small amounts urinated, bladder distention	Indication of urinary retention and stasis
Allow time to completely empty bladder when voiding	Prevents residual urine

Discharge or Maintenance Evaluation

• Urinary pattern and urine characteristics within baseline determinations
• Urine culture negative for infectious organisms
• Indwelling catheter maintained properly
• Absence of urinary symptoms indicating retention or residual

Knowledge deficit

Related to: Lack of information about prostatectomy
Defining characteristics: Request for information, anxiety about changes in sexual function, verbalization of the problem, anxiety about incontinence following surgery

Outcome Criteria

Expresses an increase in knowledge regarding temporary postoperative changes.

Interventions	Rationales
Assess presence of anxiety, concern about results of surgery and effect on lifestyle, body image	Impending surgery causes anxiety about sexual functioning and incontinence problems
Inform that postoperative incontinence is temporary and tapers off within 6 months	Incontinence caused by trauma to bladder sphincter during surgery and an indwelling catheter which reduces muscle tone
Instruct in pelvic muscle strengthening exercises to be performed for 10 minutes 4 times/day; practice starting and stopping during urination	Improves muscle tone and strength to control incontinence when stress of increased intra-abdominal pressure is present
Suggest use of pads or waterproof underwear	Prevents wetting of clothing and embarrassment

Interventions	Rationales
Suggest refraining from sexual intercourse for 3-6 weeks after surgery	Permits tissue healing
Inform of retrograde ejaculation during intercourse with transurethral prostatectomy	Prevents alarm at change in urine after intercourse and absence of semen during ejaculation
Inform about alternative sexual methods if impotency expected following prostatectomy	Provides information to allay anxiety

Discharge or Maintenance Evaluation

- Verbalizes anxiety is reduced
- Verbalizes improved understanding of consequences of surgery and possible resolution

Renal, Urinary Infections

Lower urinary tract infection (cystitis) whether acute or chronic is a common problem for both male and female elderly clients especially in the presence of an indwelling catheter. It often leads to pyelonephritis when bacteria travels up the ureters and causes infection and inflammation in the renal pelvis. Most commonly, it results from bladder neck obstruction in the male and contamination via the urethra from bowel excreta in the female.

MEDICAL CARE

Anti-infectives: amoxicillin (Amoxil); sulfisoxazole (Gantrisin); cephalexin (Keflex); gentamicin (Garamycin) PO organisms dependent to destroy and/or inhibit growth by interfering with protein synthesis

Urinary Antiseptics: methanamine mandelate (Mandelamine), nalidixic acid (NegGram) PO to treat chronic or recurrent cystitis

Analgesics: phenazopyridine (Pyridium) PO affects musoca or urinary tract to relieve pain, burning, frequency and urgency

Vitamins: ascorbic acid (Vitamin C), sodium biphosphate to acidify urine

X-ray: Kidney, ureters, bladder (HUB) reveals obstruction or other abnormality leading to UTI

Intravenous pyelogram: Reveals pathology that predisposes to obstruction or deformities of kidneys, residual urine

Ultrasound, computerized tomography: Reveals kidney abnormalities, urinary reflux

Urinalysis: Reveals large numbers of WBCs, RBCs, pus, increased pH, casts

Urine culture: Reveals increased bacterial count of more than 100,000/ml and sensitivity to specific anti-infective

CBC: Reveals increased WBC in presence of infection

NURSING CARE PLANS

Essential nursing diagnoses and plans associated with these conditions:

Altered nutrition: less than body requirements (118)

Related to: Inability to ingest food because of biological factors from acute infectious process of pyelonephritis
Defining characteristics: Nausea, vomiting, anorexia

SPECIFIC DIAGNOSES AND CARE PLANS

Pain

Related to: Biological injuring agents (infection of bladder/kidney)
Defining characteristics: Communication of pain descriptors, suprapublic, flank pain, dysuria

Outcome Criteria

Pain relieved or absent.

Renal, Urinary Infections

Aging

↓   ↓   ↓

Stasis of urine   Poor perineal hygiene   Indwelling catheter

↓

Contamination of meatus and invasion fo bladder by
Escherichia coli, Klebsiella aerobacter, Proteus mirabilis, Streptococcus facalis, Staphlococcus aureus

↓

Lower urinary tract infection

↓   ↓

Spread to ureters and renal pelvis   Cloudy, foul-smelling urine
                                                                                        Dysuria
↓   Urgency
                                                                                        Frequency
Upper urinary tract infection   Burning
(pyelonephritis)   Nocturia

↓

Flank pain
Fever, chills
Palpated kidney

Interventions	Rationales
Assess severity of pain, pain site, dysuria, burning on urination	Pain results from bladder spasms and infection; suprapubic in urinary bladder infection and flank in pyelonephritis
Administer analgesic PO depending on acuity and severity of pain	Controls pain by interfering with CNS pathways
Position with support of pillows	Promotes comfort and prevents pressure on painful area

Information, Instruction, Demonstration

Interventions	Rationales
Inform to take warm sitz baths or apply heat to perineum; avoid harsh soaps, deodorants, bath oils	Promotes comfort and relief from dysuria; use of irritating substances changes pH of perineum
Instruct to remain in close proximity to bathroom	Prevents dribbling accidents from dysuria and urgency

Discharge or Maintenance Evaluation

- Verbalizes that pain controlled
- Decreased use of analgesic

Hyperthermia

Related to: Illness (renal inflammation/infection)
Defining characteristics: Low-grade or high elevation in body temperature above normal range

Outcome Criteria

Temperature reduced to baseline level.

Interventions	Rationales
Assess temperature elevations above 96.8°F (37°C), chills, malaise, muscle aches	Systemic response to inflammation as body increases blood flow and metabolism to assist healing
Administer antipyretic	Prevents extreme elevations to protect vulnerable organs such as the brain
Administer anti-infectives specific to identified organism	Destroys organisms by inhibiting cell wall synthesis
Sponge with cool cloth with care to avoid chilling	Increases heat loss by evaporation
Provide comfortable environmental temperature; provide extra covers	Promotes comfort and prevents chilling
Increase fluid intake up to 2-3 L/day (10-12 glasses), offer ice chips, popsicles, juices of choice	Replaces fluid loss from diaphoresis and prevents dehydration
Change damp linens or clothing as needed if diaphoretic	Promotes comfort and prevents further chilling

Information, Instruction, Demonstration

Interventions	Rationales
Taking oral temperature measurement	Permits independence in monitoring temperature

Discharge or Maintenance Evaluation

- Antipyretic and/or non-medication measures effective in reducing and maintaining baseline temperature
- I&O ratio in balance
- Temperature at baseline levels within 48-72 hours

Altered patterns of urinary elimination

Related to: Mechanical trauma (renal or urinary bladder infection; use of indwelling catheter)
Defining characteristics: Dysuria, frequency, nocturia, urgency, presence of indwelling catheter for incontinence problem

Outcome Criteria

Return of normal urinary elimination patterns. Patent indwelling catheter and collection system.

Interventions	Rationales
Assess for urge incontinence, presence of cloudy, foul smelling urine voided or from catheter, urine containing pus, mucus, blood	Signs and symptoms present in renal/bladder infection as result of by-products of infection; higher incidence of UTI in elderly associated with chronic illness, immobility, neurologic changes, institutionalization
Assess changes in urinary pattern including dysuria, urgency, frequency	Result of bladder infection and spasms caused by irritation
Collect clean catch specimen and monitor urine cultures for increased colonization of bacteria	Culture revealing more than 100,000/ml indicates infection
Administer anti-infectives, sensitivity dependent	Treatment for infection specific to organism identification

Interventions	Rationales
Provide catheter care and patency by: • Preventing kinks, lying on catheter • Daily cleansing of meatal site and genitalia in females • Maintaining closed system • Maintaining collection bag below catheter insertion site • Emptying bag when two-thirds full • Avoid pulling or pressure on catheter • Using aseptic technique when obtaining specimen from catheter	Treats or prevents recurring infection via indwelling catheter
Provide access to bathroom, commode	Urgency may cause incontinence and embarrassment to client
Provide at least 2 L/day (8-10 glasses) fluids; include fruit juices	Dilutes urine and increases acidity of urine

Information, Instruction, Demonstration

Interventions	Rationales
Cleansing of genitalia and meatus after each elimination, intercourse; females wiping from front to back	Prevents contamination from genitalia
Inform to empty bladder completely and frequently and urinate when urge present	Prevents urinary stasis which creates media for bacterial growth

Discharge or Maintenance Evaluation

- Renal/bladder infection resolved with negative cultures
- Absence of urge incontinence
- Correct and appropriate administration of anti-infectives, urinary antiseptics
- Verbalizes preventive measure to take for recurrence of infection
- Catheter care and maintenance provided TID

Impotence

Aging

| ↓ | ↓ | ↓ | ↓ |

| Psychological factors | Endocrine factors | Chronic disease | Medications |
| ↓ | ↓ | ↓ | ↓ |

Chronic anxiery	Decreased secretion of	Diabetes	Antihypertensive
Depression	testosterone	COPD	Psychotrophic
Fear of loss of		Chronic renal failure	Barbituate
sexual ability		Thyroid dysfunction	Alcohol
Dependence		Vascular insufficiency	
Incontinence		Urinary diversion	
Psychic trauma		Surgical procedures on	
		reproductive organs	

| ↓ | ↓ | ↓ | ↓ |

Impotence, decreased libido

Sexual Disorders

Sexual interest and activity continue throughout life and provide physiological and psychological outlets and satisfaction for the elderly client. The intimacy of touching, closeness and sexual intercourse are expressions of sexuality that are very important to an older adult and may be altered by declining health and energy, privacy, loss of a partner, medications, chronic illness or problems of the reproductive system. Regardless of the cause, a change in sexual pattern or function results in anxiety, concern with failure and dissatisfaction with sexual intercourse which ultimately affects self-esteem, identity and role performance.

MEDICAL CARE

Estrogen: conjugated estrogen (Premarin) PO or vaginal cream as replacement therapy to relieve symptoms of dyspareunia and prevent atrophic vaginitis

Surgery: Penile transplant to maintain erection when impotence is present

NURSING CARE PLANS

Essential nursing diagnoses and plans associated with this condition:

Sexual dysfunction

Related to: Biopsychosocial alterations of sexuality - Misinformation or lack of knowledge, lack of privacy, lack of significant other, impaired relationship with significant other, altered body structure or function; drugs, surgery, disease process, radiation

Defining characteristics: Verbalization of the problem, change in sexual behavior or activities, alterations in achieving perceived sex role, actual or perceived limitation imposed by disease or therapy, alterations in achieving sexual satisfaction, inability to achieve desired satisfaction, alteration in relationship with significant other, change in interest in self and others, impotence, dyspareunia

Outcome Criteria

Adequate, satisfying sexual function.

Interventions	Rationales
Assess sexual interest, desire, affect of health status on sexuality, psychosocial factors affecting sexual function	Age related sexual changes do not alter the need for sexual closeness and companionship; however, chronic illness, drugs, fear of inability to perform, lack of or impaired relationship with partner, cultural beliefs, lack of privacy, disinterest in sex do alter sexual function
Assess presence of impotence, dyspareunia, feelings of inadequacy or fear of sexual function and failure	Changes related to aging such as slower arousal time, reduced rigidity of erection, reduced lubrication of the vagina and atrophy of vaginal lining resulting in painful intercourse may be responsible for the sexual problems; chronic illnesses compromise sexual functioning by causing physiological changes and fear of recurrence of symptoms
Include partner in discussion if appropriate; approach subject if client doesn't	May be embarrassed to have partner present or even approach the subject; may be more comfortable discussing the subject alone

Dyspareunia

Aging

↓	↓	↓
Thinning and atrophy of vaginal lining	Decreased secretion of mucus from Bartholin gland	Atrophic vaginitis
↓	↓	↓
Cracks in vaginal mucosa	Lack of vaginal lubrication	Burning Itching Infection
↓	↓	↓

Sexual dysfunction (dyspareunia)
↓

Slight bleeding from sexual intercourse
Discomfort during sexual intercourse
↓

Fear of engaging in sexual intercourse
Socialcultural influences that lead to belief that sexual activity ceases in the elderly

Interventions	Rationales
Discuss past sexual experiences and practices, interest and satisfaction, medications taken for control of chronic diseases that affect sexual function	Provides individual needs regarding sexual behavior based on history
Discuss importance to maintain sexual functioning by intercourse or masturbation	Maintains interest and sexual function
Encourage to vary positions during intercourse, pain in joints in those with arthritis, dyspnea in those with COPD, post-myocardial infarction	Pain, dyspnea may be exacerbated during exertion and a more passive position and participation promotes safe sexual activity
Provide privacy, warm shower or bath; avoidance of large meals or excessive alcohol before sexual activity	Some elderly live with family members or in long-term facilities and may lack the privacy needed because of attitudes about aging and sex
Provide pain medication, bronchodilators, oxygen, vasodilators as appropriate to illness before sexual intercourse	Promotes comfort, prevents pain, dyspnea during activity as pulse, BP, and 0_2 consumption increase
Use exercise and pain tolerance, changes in VS caused by activity, as guidelines for a progressive sexual activity plan based on physical limits	Provides baselines for plan to promote sexual activity without symptoms that create fear or interfere with sexual activity

Information, Instruction, Demonstration

Interventions	Rationales
Correct any misinformation about effects of sexual activity; inform client that correct information assists to identify fears, concerns and remedy sexual dysfunction	Fear of precipitating angina episode, heart attack, dyspnea from COPD, injury to inflamed joints usually caused by lack of correct information
Inform of age-related physical changes, male/female reproductive system (anatomy and physiology), four phases of the intercourse cycle for male/female	Provides information to promote understanding of sexual functioning
Inform to avoid sexual activity if environmental temperature is excessively hot or cold, after eating large meal, if anxious or angry or fatigued	Has a negative effect on sexual ability and activity
If partner recently died, inform of importance of continuing sexual activity	A loss of sexual functioning may occur with prolonged abstinence
Inform of erectile or ejaculation changes related to disease or surgery; retrograde ejaculation causing a cloudy appearance to the urine, impotence from erectile or ejaculation failure, effect of fear on libido	Reduces anxiety and fear of impotence; change in urine in diabetes and following transurethral prostatectomy caused by incomplete closure of bladder sphincter, circulatory impairment in diabetes or atherosclerosis affecting blood flow and interfering with ability to achieve an erection
Inform of effect of drugs on sexual performance; suggest discussion with physician about problem	The changing, elimination or adjustments in doses of medications may prevent or reduce impotence

Interventions	Rationales
Use charts to demonstrate position variations for arthritic, stroke, COPD, MI, angina clients; instruct in use of medications, warm application, when to cease activity and rest	More dependent, passive positions permits intercourse without producing symptoms that interfere with performance
Instruct female client to use water-soluble lubricant during intercourse	Lubricants vagina to prevent pain and irritation during intercourse from thinning, dry mucosa
Inform of penile implant possibility and to discuss with physician	Treatment for impotence caused by stroke or surgery that does not respond to therapy
Instruct female with catheter to tape to thigh or abdomen; male to hold catheter in place with condom and tape tubing to abdomen. Catheter should be disconnected from tubing and clamped	Stabilizes catheter and prevents injury to the urethra, backflow is prevented by clamp
If incontinent of feces, instruct to administer enema before intercourse	Decreases possibility of fecal incontinence during intercourse
Instruct to void before and after intercourse	Clears meatus of infectious organisms that may cause bladder infection
Suggest sexual or psychological therapy if appropriate to enhance appearance and increase desirability	Anxiety and reduced self-esteem resulting from altered sexuality are common problems that can be helped by counseling

Interventions	Rationales
If sexual dysfunction a result of cognitive functioning, inform family of reduced sex interest and inappropriate sexual behaviors	Promotes understanding of antisocial sexual behavior as dementia progresses and prevents embarrassment to family

Discharge or Maintenance Evaluation

- Verbalizes sexuality changes associated with aging
- Verbalizes difficulties, limitations of sexual experience and possible reasons for them
- VS within baseline ranges after intercourse
- Identification, maintenance of desired sexual activity
- Verbalizes satisfaction with alteration in sexual patterns and sexual intercourse alterations within physical limitations
- Reduced anxiety and fear in contemplation of intercourse
- Return to previous sexual patterns as a result of rehabilitation
- Absence of discomfort during intercourse
- Proper use of medications and other preparations before intercourse
- Measures taken to reduce inappropriate sexual behavior by mentally incapacitated elderly
- Appropriate environment established for optimal sexual functioning
- Expression of reduced anxiety as sexual activity improves

Urinary Elimination Disorders

Urinary incontinence is the involuntary loss of urine. Although normal aging is not considered a cause of incontinence, frequency of this condition does increase as one ages. It is usually the result of physical health (immobility, changes in muscle tone, infection, neuropathology) or mental health (cognitive, intellectual deficits). Chronic incontinence, regardless of the amount of urine lost or if continual, is dependent on the maintenance of the urine storage and expulsion processes which are the basis for urine continence. Its affect on an elderly client includes loss of self-esteem and independence, social isolation, depression, fear and anxiety. Urinary diversion is a surgical procedure associated with the removal of the total, partial, or a segment of the urinary bladder. It is usually performed to treat malignancy but can also be done to establish urinary drainage in those with spinal cord injury (neurogenic bladder), obstructive conditions, severe and persistent cystitis with hemorrhage, or trauma of the lower tract preventing normal function. Types of diversion include a cutaneous ureterostomy or a vesicostomy and formation of a stoma. Drainage of urine from these procedures can be accomplished by intermittent catheterization. Another procedure is the ileal conduit (most common procedure) in which the ureters are implanted into the terminal ileum and a portion is brought to the skin surface and stoma formed. Urine flows into the conduit developed by the bowel and urinary elimination takes place by intestinal peristalsis that empties into an appliance and collecting system fitted over the stoma.

MEDICAL CARE

Cholinergics: bethanechol chloride (Urecholine) PO to contract detrusor muscle of the urinary bladder to encourage urination

Anticholinergics: propantheline bromide (Probanthine) PO to increase bladder capacity, and relieve urgency, frequency, dysuria and nocturia

Antispasmodics: oxybutynin (Ditropan) PO to reduce bladder spasms and flavoxate (Urispas) PO to relieve inflammation of urethra, bladder, prostate gland

Alpha-adrenergic blockers: prazosin (Minipress) PO to relax spastic bladder neck

Cystometry: Measures volume-pressure relationship and may be used as a therapeutic exercise to improve bladder capacity and increase control of the voiding reflex

Urinalysis: Reveals any abnormal constituents in urine (blood, glucose, protein), urine culture to reveal presence of urinary bladder infection if bacterial count over 100,000/ml

Surgery: Implanted artificial sphincter at urethral site with an inflatable cuff that surrounds proximal urethral which is connected to a tubing and in implanted fluid reservoir and an inflation bulb; pressing the bulb inflates the cuff and prevents passage of urine

NURSING CARE PLANS

Essential nursing diagnoses and plans associated with this condition:

Risk for impaired skin integrity (246)

Related to: External factors of excretions from incontinence or urine
Defining characteristics: Reddened, irritated skin at perineal and buttocks area, disruption of skin surface, excoriation, maceration of exposed skin

Sleep pattern disturbance (77)

Related to: Internal factors from illness
Defining characteristics: Interrupted sleep, nocturia, verbal complaints of not feeling well rested

Urinary Incontinence

Aging

↓   ↓   ↓   ↓

Dementia Confusion	Decreased bladder muscle tone and weakness of pelvic muscles and urethral sphincter Prostatectomy Urinary tract infection	Reduced bladder size and capacity Bladder overdistention, retention Bladder irritation, spasms (infection) Indwelling catheter CNS depressant drugs	Sensory, cognitive or mobility deficits Neurological dysfunction Neuropathy affecting awareness of bladder fullness Spinal cord nerve injury/disease

↓   ↓   ↓   ↓

Unaware of need to urinate Inability to make effort to urinate	Bladder pressure exceeds maximal urethral pressure in absence of detrusor activity	Strong desire to urinate	Absence of sensation and desire to urinate Unpredictable urination Unawareness of incontinence Constant flow of urine Loss of urine before reaching bathroom

      ↓   ↓   ↓

Psychological incontinence	Increased intra-abdominal pressure	Inability to reach bathroom on time	

      ↓   ↓

	Activity causing pressure on bladder (coughing, laughing, lifting, climbing stairs)	Urge incontinence Overflow incontinence	Functional incontinence Total incontinence

      ↓

Stress incontinence

Altered thought processes (70)

Related to: Physiological changes, psychological conflicts, impaired judgement, loss of memory
Defining characteristics: Cognitive, memory deficit, disorientation, depression

Functional incontinence (154)

Related to: Sensory, cognitive or mobility deficits from aging changes
Defining characteristics: Unaware of need to urinate, absence of sensation and desire to urinate, inability to reach bathroom in time

SPECIFIC DIAGNOSES AND CARE PLANS

Chronic low self-esteem

Related to: Biophysical, psychosocial factors (incontinence)
Defining characteristics: Self-neglecting verbalization, expressions of shame/guilt, embarrassment about incontinence, evaluates self as unable to deal with events, progressive dependent behavior

Outcome Criteria

Improved self-esteem.

Interventions	Rationales
Assess feelings about loss of ability to control urination, effect on appearance and socialization, ability to use devices to control incontinence	Provides information about effects of incontinence on self-esteem, body image

Interventions	Rationales
Assess presence of indwelling catheter and use of leg bag	Leg bag allows for mobility and socialization
Provide protective pads or garments (disposable)	Protects clothing, seats from moisture causing embarrassment
Allow to express feelings in a warm, non-threatening, non-judgmental environment	Reduces anxiety and promotes trust

Information, Instruction, Demonstration

Interventions	Rationales
Inform about devices available to control incontinence	Self-esteem enhanced if continence established or incontinence controlled
Suggest support group (Help for Incontinent People); use of biofeedback technique	Provides information and support to eliminate or cope with problem

Discharge or Maintenance Evaluation

- Verbalizes improved self-esteem with increased information and use of aids to control incontinence
- Absence of isolation; increased social involvement
- Involvement in support group if appropriate
- Uses techniques to improve appearance and continence

Risk for infection

Related to: Invasive procedure (indwelling catheter)
Defining characteristics: Catherization (intermittent) or indwelling catheter in place, elevated temperature,

low fluid intake, failure to remove soiled protective pads or garments, use of continent aids, urinary retention, stasis, cloudy, foul smelling urine voided or via catheter, urinary, frequency, burning on urination

Outcome Criteria

Absence of urinary bladder infection.

Interventions	Rationales
Assess need for, presence of cateterization/ indwelling catheter, type of drainage, urine characteristics	Catherization is only done as a last resort and indwelling catheter insertion is done for total incontinence or in cases where continence rehabilitation has proved ineffective
Collect mid-stream urine or remove from closed urinary system with sterile needle and syringe for culture	Identifies type and number of colonizations of microorganisms if infection present
Use sterile technique in catheter care, handwashing before catheter care procedures	Prevents transmission of infectious agents via catheter
Provide daily intake of up to 2 L	Dilutes urine and reduces risk for bladder infection
Maintain closed urinary drainage system properly: • Prevent kinks or lying on tubing • Place tubing lower than catheter insertion site; tape to leg • Maintain closed system; empty from bottom of bag when two-thirds full	Prevent back flow and contamination of urine

Information, Instruction, Demonstration

Interventions	Rationales
Demonstrate and instruct in self-catherization using sterile technique if appropriate	Promotes continence and independence

Discharge or Maintenance Evaluation

- Absence of urinary bladder infection
- Proper clean and sterile techniques performed as preventive measures in catheter insertion and/or care
- Indwelling catheter patency and sterility maintained

Altered patterns of urinary elimination

Related to: Sensory motor, neuromuscular impairment, mechanical trauma (urinary incontinence)
Defining characteristics: Incontinence, urgency, frequency, cognitive, mobility deficits, bladder overdistention, nocturia, bladder spasms, inability to reach bathroom in time, catheterization

Outcome Criteria

Restoration of or optimal urinary continence potential.

Interventions	Rationales
Assess suprapubic area for distention, urgency frequency, nocturia, dysuria, amount of urine loss with each incontinence episode or if continuous, recent removal of catheter	Provides information regarding functional abnormalities of urinary system, extent of incontinence problem

Interventions	Rationales
Assess presence of chronic illness, urinary tract infection, indwelling catheter	Predisposes client to incontinence; diabetes, CVA, Parkinson's are chronic illnesses associated with bladder dysfunction
Assess cognitive and mobility deficiencies	Awareness of need to urinate and ability to reach bathroom necessary to prevent incontinence
Offer opportunity for voiding q2h or schedule according to baseline patterns	Promotes and reminds of voiding to prevent urine loss
Allow to sit upright or stand to urinate	Promotes urination by gravity in accustomed position
Alter environment with raised seats on toilet, holding bars, clear pathways	Provides easy access to facilities and use of toilet if mobility deficit exists
Provide clothing that is easy to manipulate for toileting	Promotes independence and ease of exposure for urination
Provide slight pressure on bladder, allowing water to run, stroking of skin above pubis	Aids in urination by sensory stimulation
Provide urinary rehabilitation or training by providing scheduled elimination during day and night and gradually lengthen interval between voidings	Restores urinary continence if physical cause; modifies behavior if psychological cause of incontinence
Provide penile clamp or external condom	Noncatheter devices for males that obstruct urine flow or collect urine as it flows

Interventions	Rationales
Provide urinary collection device and attach over perineal area • Noncatheter device for women that collects urine as it flows • Catheterize or insert indwelling catheter if appropriate	Provides collection of urine if all other methods fail
Provide battery-operated electrodes that contract pelvic floor muscles	Occludes bladder outlet in males and females
Provide protective pads for females and dribbling bag for males; protective undergarments for both depending on amount of urinary loss	Absorbs or collects urine when incontinence cannot be prevented

Information, Instruction, Demonstration

Interventions	Rationales
Inform of alternative methods available to control or collect urine flow; protective pads or garments	Offers client opportunity to select best device or protection
Instruct in Kegel exercises and frequency in performance each day	Strengthens pelvic muscles in females
Instruct in effect of drugs on potential for incontinence	Increases awareness of possible changes in patterns if taking diuretics or sedatives or psychotrophics
Assist to plan a schedule of ADL that includes regular urination opportunities	Promotes continence

Interventions	Rationales
Instruct in fluid intake over 24 hours that coincides with urinary schedule	Promotes continence and prevents accidents
Instruct in intermittent catheterization technique	Possible for a select group of clients
Instruct in cleansing and care of devices if appropriate, removing and reapplying	Prevents infection of urinary tract

Discharge or Maintenance Evaluation

- Restoration of continence urinary pattern or reduction in number of incontinent episodes
- Ability to use and care for urinary devices and protective garments
- Follows bladder training schedule successfully
- Performs daily exercises to strengthen perineal and sphincter muscles
- Performs self-catheterization if appropriate
- Uses alternate methods to control incontinence
- Environment and clothing modifications to facilitate continence
- Absence of urinary tract infection from use of urinary devices, protective garments, improper perineal care after voiding

Knowledge deficit

Related to: Lack of general care information about ostomy procedures, intermittent self-catheterization, measures to prevent complications
Defining characteristics: Request for information about urinary diversion care

Outcome Criteria

Ability to perform appropriate care of urinary diversion

Interventions	Rationales
Pathophysiology and urinary diversion anatomic changes, type of ostomy, characteristics of urinary output	Provides information and rationale for functional pattern of urinary elimination
Dressing change and stoma protection during bathing, cleanse peri-stomal area with mild soap and warm water, gently pat dry	Maintains clean, dry stoma and per-stomal skin; cleanses secretions or debris from peristomal skin
Removal and application of appliance, pouch application and emptying when 1/3 full, empty bag as appropriate, associated skin and stoma care with barrier or sealant to protect from irritation and breakdown	Ensures proper and safe care and use of ostomy supplies
Proper cleansing of pouches, use of deodorant tablets in pouch	Minimizes embarrassing odors from long-term use or reused pouch
Intermittent self-catheterization of vesicostomy q3-4h, care and preparation of catheters for future	Ensures removal of urine at appropriate times from pouch created to hold urine
Inform that stoma size will reach permanent status by 4 months	Prevents anxiety caused by changes in stoma
Fluid intake of 2 to 3 L/day spread over 24 hours to include acidic liquids	Ensures adequate fluid intake to dilute urine, encourage output, and lower pH to prevent infection
Suggest alternative sexual activities, covering stoma during sexual activity, possibility of sexuality counseling	Assistive aids can enhance sexual satisfaction

Interventions	Rationales
Report any redness, swelling, or pain at stoma site, change in urinary pattern, output, characteristics, temperature elevation, stoma changes	Signs and symptoms of possible complications of urinary diversion

Discharge or Maintenance Evaluation

- Performs care of stoma, peristomal skin, self-catheterization, appliance removal and application
- Requests assistance and/or asks questions when needed
- Maintains adequate daily fluid intake
- Reports any signs and symptoms of urinary infection, changes in stoma or peristomal site

Musculoskeletal System

Musculoskeletal System

Including the most visible changes present in the aging person, the musculoskeletal system is concerned with body movement, posture, stability, coordination and muscular agility, strength and endurance. Neuromuscular function changes also contribute to alterations in movement as a result of peripheral motor neurons, myoneural synapses and central nervous system influences. The most distressing complaint from problems related to this system is the effect on a client's lifestyle by causing difficulty in maintaining self-care in activities of daily living. Although the elderly tend to feel that musculoskeletal disorders are inevitable and irreversible, rehabilitation has successfully restored clients to their former capabilities or assisted them in making the most of existing capabilities

GENERAL MUSCULOSKELETAL CHANGES ASSOCIATED WITH THE AGING PROCESS

Structural changes

- Loss of muscle fiber causing wasting of skeletal muscle
- Increased muscle wasting causing decreased muscle weight, strength and limitation in mobility
- Decreased muscle mass causing changes in strength, endurance and agility
- Loss of bone minerals and mass with wasting of muscles causing brittle bones, postural changes and potential for fractures
- Loss of bone mass, subcutaneous fat causing bony appearance with a prominent forehead, sunken eyes
- Stretching of ligaments causing joint stiffness and reduced motion
- Kyphosis of dorsal spine, shortening of vertebral column, hip and knee flexion causing postural changes and reduced height
- Postural changes causing center of gravity change from middle of hips to chest area affecting body balance and potential for falls

Physiologic changes

- Altered circulatory and respiratory function (O_2 supply) causing decreased muscle activity
- Decreased storage of muscle glycogen causing loss of energy needed for increased activity
- Change in extrapyramidal system causing muscle stiffness, slowness and resting tremor
- Resorption in bone faster than formation of new bone causing potential for fracture
- Changes in enzyme function causing muscle fatigue
- Increased fragility of synovial membranes and thickness of fluid causing joint changes
- Decreased motor coordination and manual skills causing decreased reaction time
- Increased muscle cramping and paresthesias of the legs (restless legs) causing pain, sleep deprivation
- Weakened bone, muscle changes, change in center of gravity causing falls
- Long time stress of weight bearing on feet causing mechanical and dermatological changes and foot disabilities

ESSENTIAL NURSING DIAGNOSES AND CARE PLANS

Impaired physical mobility

Related to: Intolerance to activity; decreased strength and endurance
Defining characteristics: Decreased muscle strength, control and/or mass, inability to purpose-fully move within physical environment including bed mobility, transfer and ambulation

Related to: Pain and discomfort
Defining characteristics: Reluctance to attempt movement, limited range of motion, imposed restrictions of movement, including mechanical; medical protocol, inability to purposefully move within physical environment, including bed mobility, transfer and ambulation

Related to: Perceptual or cognitive impairment
Defining characteristics: Mentation, level of consciousness, neurosensory deficit, inability to purposefully move within physical environment, including bed mobility, transfer and ambulation

Related to: Neuromuscular impairment
Defining characteristics: Paresthesias, paralysis, impaired coordination, gait disturbances, balancing problems, decreased muscle control, inability to purposefully move within physical environment including bed mobility, transfer and ambulation

Related to: Musculoskeletal impairment
Defining characteristics: Inability to purposefully move within physical environment including bed mobility, transfer and ambulation, reluctance to attempt movement, imposed restriction of movement, including medical protocol, mechanical; fracture, foot disorders, arthritis, peripheral vascular disease

Related to: Depression, severe anxiety
Defining characteristics: Reluctance to attempt movement, low energy level, fear of falling, confusion, stress, impaired judgement

Outcome Criteria

Return to and/or maintenance of baseline mobility and performance of ADL within physical/mental limitations.

Interventions	Rationales
Assess activity level, ability to move in bed, ambulate, perform ADL and amount of assistance needed, degree and type of mobility impairment	Assists to determine the activities to eliminate, what assistance is needed, measures to take to protect and preserve existing muscle, skeletal function
Assess muscle weakness, atrophy, tone, presence of skeletal contractures, deformities	Provides information of existing muscle function and potential for optimal functional achievement
Assess for pain in joints or bone pain, joint movement and stability, foot discomfort when ambulating, ability to perform active ROM, presence of fracture	Pain prevents optimal mobility effort and may indicate need for imposed immobility to prevent injury to joints or bone fracture
Perform active, passive or assistive active ROM as appropriate	Promotes joint mobility and prevents contractures
Apply dry or moist heat to muscles; massage muscles if appropriate	Relaxes muscles and reduces muscle spasms causing pain
Position in proper body alignment including extremities that are affected by neuromuscular or musculoskeletal impairment	Maintains anatomical position and preserves functional ability
Provide pillows, sand bags, trochanter rolls, slings for support as appropriate	Promotes comfort, maintains proper position, prevents pressure and edema of body part
Move or reposition gently and carefully, maintain joint on paralyzed side higher than joint proximal to it	Prevents tension or pressure on affected part
Monitor VS before and after activity, cease activity if sudden change present (dyspnea, increased BP and P)	Provides data regarding cardiac status

Interventions	Rationales
Utilize foot board, hand rolls, boot on feet (soft devices preferable)	Prevents contractures of hand or feet, flexion deformities or sublixation or hypertonia of fingers
Assist to perform ADL as needed; identify activities that can be performed independently and give positive reinforcement for attempts	Maintains as much independence as possible and improves self-esteem
Provide assistive aids (cane, walker, holding bars, bed pulls, trapeze, gait and transfer belts)	Assists in mobility while preventing accidents
Limit positioning on an affected part of body to 1 hour	Prevents compromised lung expansion and circulation to part

Information, Instruction, Demonstration

Interventions	Rationales
Instruct in quadricep sitting and gluteal sitting exercises	Strengthens muscles and prepares them for ambulation
Instruct to initiate ambulation by: • Applying brace if appropriate • Sitting up in bed or on edge of bed • Assist to change positions from sitting to lying, lying to sitting, moving from bed to chair, sitting to standing • Checking balance when standing	Beginning rehabilitation and activity program when not in therapy that can be incorporated into daily care

Interventions	Rationales
• Assisting to walk using parallel bars or walker or 3 or 4 legged cane as appropriate if arms can be used	
Step-by-step instruction in active ROM, positioning of affected limbs during sleep, transfer techniques, use of unaffected side to assist in climbing stairs or transferring	Promotes independence and mobility
Continue physical therapy and schedule to perform activities	Promotes continuity of care and successful rehabilitation
Suggest occupational therapy if appropriate	Provides retraining in fine motor activity
Provide information in use of hand rails, ambulatory aids	Prevents accidental falls
Demonstrate application of leg brace or splints to arm	Provides support for affected limb
Procedure for sitting in and getting up from chair that is raised and has arms	Promotes independence in performing procedures
Inform to step over imaginary or real line on floor, lift toes when stepping, rock back and forth, take a step backward and two forward	Measures to relieve bradykinesia when freezing occurs in neuromuscular disorder
Carry article in hands, put hands in pocket	Decreases tremor and/or embarrassment
Instruct in exercise modification for client in wheelchair	Instruct in exercise modification for client in wheelchair

Interventions	Rationales
Instruct in safety measures in environment, placing articles within reach	Prevents falls during ambulation or from reaching
Instruct in individual exercise program and need for proper monitoring and supervision; to avoid isometric exercises (increase BP) and to increase exercises slowly	Exercises benefit self-esteem, improve digestion, respirations, cardiovascular functions, increase coping ability and stress reduction

Discharge or Maintenance Evaluation

- Absence of contractures
- Continues motor function at optimal level
- Maintains optimal independence in mobility within limitations imposed by disease
- Participates in daily exercise, physical therapy program
- Utilizes aids to facilitate movement
- Absence of falls or injury to affected extremities
- Able to sit up, lie down, transfer to chair, stand
- Progressive adaptation to neuromuscular deficits

Risk for trauma

Related to: Internal factors — Weakness, poor vision, temperature/tactile sensation, balancing difficulties, reduced muscle (large or small) coordination, handeye coordination, lack of safety education, precautions, cognitive or emotional difficulties
Defining characteristics: Tripping, stumbling, repeated falls, sudden injury, trauma, fracture, disorientation, mentation problems, muscle, joint pain, loss of tone, calcium absorption, restraining practices, poor supervision, personal physical assault, abuse, altered mobility

Related to: External factors unsafe environment
Defining characteristics: Wet floors, cluttered pathways, unanchored rugs, poor lighting, absent hand rails, mobility aids, too hot or cold water for bathing or treatments, not using visual or auditory aids, fracture/trauma from falls, multiple medications

Outcome Criteria

Absence of trauma, injury, fracture, falls.

Interventions	Rationales
Assess mobility and stability, muscle weakness, cognitive limitations, balance or gait difficulties	Falls common in elderly and result from weakness in muscle and skeletal support system
Assess sensory deficits of visual, tactile, perceptual changes	Contributes to falls and other trauma because of insensitivity to hot/cold, pain
Assess changes in mentation, vertigo, syncope, wandering	Provides information regarding potential for falls/trauma
Assess for unexplained injury, protective behavior, excessive fear, repeated trauma	May indicate physical abuse
Assess environment for safety hazards; lighting, pathways, absence of aids, high beds, articles out of reach	Predisposes to falls, injury
Provide low bed, side rails if appropriate; place mattress near floor if danger of falling	Protects from falls
Provide night light, clear pathways, dry, non-slippery floor	Prevents bumping into objects or stumbling and falling
Provide assistance in ambulation, assistive aids as needed	Promotes safety and prevents falls if too weak or impaired to walk alone
Remain if complains of feeling dizzy or faint	Reduces anxiety. potential injury from fall when fainting
Apply alarm system to alert that wandering outside of safe limits	Allows wandering a safe distance rather than use of restraints or other confinement method

Interventions	Rationales
Allow for and encourage safe activities when scheduled or desired	Promotes socialization

Information, Instruction, Demonstration

Interventions	Rationales
Instruct in environmental modification that accommodates level of functioning and awareness	Creates safe environment and prevents injury
Refrain from driving if not capable	Cognitive difficulties may cause injury to client and/or others
Instruct in risk factors associated with falls and fractures (diseases that affect mobility and thought processes)	Provides information to reinforce compliance in preventing injury
Instruct in side effects of medications being taken and potential for causing falls	Promotes understanding of effect medications have on well-being or injury
Instruct to change positions slowly	Orthostatic hypotension causes dizziness and possible fainting resulting in fall
Advise to wear supportive, sturdy shoes with broad heels	Prevents slipping, stumbling

Discharge or Maintenance Evaluation

- Absence of falls or injury from dangerous objects
- Safety hazards removed
- Wandering within safe environment
- Ambulates safely with assistance or use of aids Arthritis

Osteoarthritis

Aging (long-term trauma)

↓

Alteration in chondrocyte function in movable joints

↓   ↓

Cartilage softening, yellowish color   Alteration in subchondral bone

↓   ↓

Fissures and pitting of joint   Sclerosis or formation of new bone near a joint

↓   ↓

Diffuse ulceration of joint   Cyst formation

↓   ↓

Cartilage erosion   Osteophyte spur formation

↓   ↓

Cartillage thinning and destruction to the bone

↓   ↓

Aching pain at joints (hands, feet, hips, knees, cervical vertebrae)
Stiffness of joints especially in AM
Crepitus on movement
Joint enlargement
Limited movement of joint
Synovitis

Arthritis

Osteoarthritis is a degenerative noninflammatory arthritic disorder of the joints; rheumatoid arthritis is a systemic inflammatory disease of the joints. Both are chronic debilitating diseases leading to deformities and progressive mobility and activity impairment. Joints most commonly affected by osteoarthritis are the hips, knees, cervical, thoracic and lumbar; by rheumatoid arthritis are hands, feet, arms and knees

MEDICAL CARE

Nonopoid Analgesics/Nonsteroid anti-inflammatories: ibuprofen (Motrin), indomethacin (Indocin), aspirin PO to inhibit prostaglandin biosynthesis in treatment of arthritis

Corticosteroids: prednisone (Deltasone) PO, prednisolone tebutate (Hydeltra) intrasynovial as an anti-inflammatory to treat rheumatoid arthritis

Immunosuppressants: azathioprine (Imuran) PO to treat rheumatoid arthritis that is unresponsive to conventional therapy to modify the disease process

Antirheumatics: aurothioglucose (Solganal) IM gold compound to suppress inflammatory process in joint by suppressing immune response used for rheumatoid arthritis

Antigout agent: Colchicine PO to decrease pain and inflammation in acute gouty arthiritis and prevent recurrent attacks

X-ray of joints: Reveals joint space narrowing, osteophyte formation and subchondral bony sclerosis and cyst formation in osteoarthritis; bone destruction in osteoarthritis; joint space narrowing, destruction of articular cartilage, erosion and deformity in rheumatoid arthritis

Synovial fluid analysis: Reveals cloudy appearance, increased WBCs, decreased complement components in presence of rheumatoid arthritis

Rheumatoid factor (RF): Reveals presence of factor in some clients with rheumatoid arthritis

Erythrocyte sedimentation (ESR): Reveals increases in presence of inflammation

Surgical procedures: Joint replacement, synovectomy and possibly arthrodesis

NURSING CARE PLANS

Essential nursing diagnoses and plans associated with these conditions:

Impaired physical mobility (196)

Related to: Pain and discomfort and musculoskeletal impairment and limited range of motion from joint and cartilage dysfunction and disease
Defining characteristics: Joint pain, swelling, stiffness, limited movement and function of joint

Risk for impaired skin integrity (246)

Related to: External mechanical factor of pressure from splints
Defining characteristics: Irritation or disruption of skin surface underneath appliance

SPECIFIC DIAGNOSES AND CARE PLANS

Chronic pain

Related to: Chronic physical disability (decreased joint movement and stability, inflammatory process)
Defining characteristics: Verbal report of pain experienced for more than 6 months, altered ability to continue previous activities, guarded movement, stiffness of joints, joint warmth, redness, swelling

Outcome Criteria

Relief or control of pain in affected joints.

Interventions	Rationales
Assess for pain descriptors, aching and stiffness of joints especially in morning, pain on movement of joints	Results from inflammation and destructive process caused by the disease
Administer analgesic, anti-inflammatory agents	Reduces inflammation causing pain and provides relief from pain
Apply moist or dry heat or cold to painful areas (packs, heat lamp, wax baths, heating pad)	Reduces pain by use of cold if joint warm or during an acute attack of inflammation to prevent damage to joint; moist heat to treat subacute states to relieve pain
Apply splint, offer use of assistive aids	Immobilizes and protects joint to reduce pain on movement and allows for self-care activities independently

Information, Instruction, Demonstration

Interventions	Rationales
Inform of principles of joint protection and pain reduction (use of assistive devices when indicated, avoid positions of stress and joint deviation, avoid tasks that cause pain, avoid forceful and repetitive movements, perform tasks in less stressful ways and develop pacing techniques)	Protects joint while reducing pain

Interventions	Rationales
Inform of importance of compliance in taking analgesic, anti-inflammatory medications	Controls pain and inflammation
Inform of availability of non-pharmacological techniques (relaxation, biofeedback, transcutaneous electrical nerve stimulation, resting joints)	Reduces pain according to client desires
Inform to report side effects of medication regimen (rash, nausea, vomiting, bleeding from gastrointestinal tract)	Drug toxicity common in the elderly as renal clearance is decreased

Discharge or Maintenance Evaluation

- Periods of pain relief and control
- Compliance with medication regimen to control pain
- Compliance with methods to protect joints from pain and damage

Ineffective individual coping

Related to: Multiple life changes (limitations imposed on lifestyle by disease)
Defining characteristics: Inability to meet role expectations, inability to meet basic needs, alteration in societal participation, chronic fatigue, chronic worry

Related to: Inadequate coping method
Defining characteristics: Inability to problem. solve, poor self-esteem, chronic anxiety

Outcome Criteria

Adaptation to chronic, disabling disesase with optimal adjustments in lifestyle in relation to physical activities.

Interventions	Rationales
Assess use of coping skills, ability to cope with fear associated with changes in mobility/activity pattern and fatigue, chronicity of worry and anxiety	Older adults display outstanding ability to cope and adapt, although inability to maintain independence and control over life leads to frustration and negative feelings about lifestyle
Assist to identify positive defense mechanisms and promote behaviors to be learned	Use of defense mechanisms that have worked in past increases ability to cope and promotes self-esteem

Information, Instruction, Demonstration

Interventions	Rationales
Provide environment that allows for free expression of concerns and fears	Encourages trust and relieves anxiety
Social and coping skills with problem-solving approaches	Prevents disengagement and promotes coping ability with lifestyle changes
Relaxation techniques	Reduces anxiety and stress associated with decreasing functional abilities
New ways or methods to adapt roles to new situation or needs	Provides for alternatives that increase participation and independence in activities
Suggest psychotherapy or support group if appropriate	Provides variety of techniques to reduce anxiety and stress

Discharge or Maintenance Evaluation

- Uses appropriate coping and problem-solving skills in adapting to functional losses
- Level of independence appropriate for functional ability
- Asks for assistance when needed
- Verbalization of reduced anxiety and fear
- Participation in social activities according to preference and activity tolerance

Body image disturbance

Related to: Biophysical factors (deformed joints)
Defining characteristics: Verbal response to actual change in structure and/or function, negative feelings about body/deformities, physical change caused by disease (deformities)

Outcome Criteria

Enhanced body image with adaptation to use of splints, assistive aids or measures to function with impaired mobility and joint function.

Interventions	Rationales
Assess for expression of feelings about appearance, effect on lifestyle, socializing activities	Provides information about effect on body image and ability to adapt to and manage changes
Assist to recognize limited function, loss of self-esteem and anxiety and fear about deformity and disabilities	Promotes identification of normal reactions and concerns associated with losses and change in chronic illness
Provide psychological support in non-threatening environment	Promotes trusting and effective relationship needed for compliance

Information, Instruction, Demonstration

Interventions	Rationales
Offer suggestions of clothing to purchase that will cover deformity and/or splint	Promotes body image
Suggest support group or counseling (Arthritis Foundation)	Provides information, equipment and support

Discharge or Maintenance Evaluation

- Improved body image by change in clothing and appearance
- Modifies lifestyle to improve self-esteem and body image
- Expression of feelings about disability and functional changes
- Statements that ability and confidence have increased in dealing with deformities and disabilities

Self-care deficit: bathing, hygiene, dressing, grooming, feeding

Related to: Impaired mobility status, pain, musculoskeletal impairment (limited joint movement, loss of function

Defining characteristics: Inability to wash body or body parts, inability to put on or take off clothing and fasten it, inability to feed self without assistance, inability to maintain appearance at satisfactory level

Outcome Criteria

Appropriately bathed, groomed, dressed and fed independently or with assistance of aids.

Interventions	Rationales
Assess ability for self-care in performing ADL, ability to use articles for washing, grooming and eating, specific deficits	Provides information regarding needs and amount of assistance needed; joint pain and mobility may be continuous or intermittent and imposed rest of joints may be necessary if inflammation present
Allow time to perform each task; avoid rushing or adhering to a schedule	Promotes self-care and avoids frustration
Provide clothing with velcro fasteners, zippers, elastic waist on clothing, front closings	Enhances dressing self if unable to manipulate buttons and ties
Provide large handled cups, eating utensils; pour liquids and cut meats if needed	Promotes self-feeding and independence
Provide assistive aids in walking (cane, walker)	Provides means to get to bathing facilities
Provide articles and aids to comb hair, brush teeth, put on makeup, built up seats	Reduces stress on joints by using aids for all self-care procedures

Information, Instruction, Demonstration

Interventions	Rationales
Schedule to organize tasks	Prevents excessive use of joints
Instruct in use of aids and performing tasks slowly and in a step-by-step process	Assists to ease anxiety in use of devices and simplifies tasks

Discharge or Maintenance Evaluation

- Participation in ADL within limitations
- Accepts assistance when necessary
- Utilizes assistive aids when performing ADL
- Prevents stress on joints when performing self-care

Fractures, Trauma

Aging

↓   ↓   ↓

Osteoporosis, tumors   Fall, trauma   Abuse, neglect
↓   ↓   ↓

Pathological fracture   Sudden injury   ←
↓   ↓   ↓

Bone fracture   ←   Unsafe environment
↓   Inadequate supervision
                                                                      Restraining practices
Pain, swelling   Assault on client
Loss of function   ↓
Abnormal movement
Deformity   Falls/injury
                                                                      Unexplained bruises or fractures

Fractures, Trauma

Falls are greatly feared in the elderly population because the incidence of falls that result in fractures increase with age. Risk factors associated with fractures/trauma in the elderly are loss of muscle tone, muscle weakness, changes in gait and balance, environmental hazards, neurosensory deficits, neuromuscular deficits, multiple medication administration and diseases such as osteoporosis, foot disorders, peripheral vascular disease, cerebrovascular accident, arthritis. A newer area of concern involving trauma in the elderly is physical abuse or neglect which results in injury because of assault or physical violence against an elderly client or failure to provide a safe environment. Both constitute a threat to the well-being of elderly clients that are not able or are too intimidated to defend themselves. Types of falls are: premonitory as a result of tripping or stumbling, drop attacks which occur as a result of loss of consciousness without warning for an unknown reason, falling which is the result of multiple falls from physical or mental impairment/diseases

MEDICAL CARE

Analgesics: acetaminophen (Tylenol), oxycodone (Percodan) PO or meperidine (Demerol) IM depending on severity of pain

X-ray: Reveals fracture site and type of fracture

Electrolyte panel: Reveals presence of any deficiencies, dehydration

CBC: Reveals presence of anemia or infection

NURSING CARE PLANS

Essential nursing diagnoses and plans associated with these conditions:

Impaired physical mobility (196)

Related to: Pain, discomfort and musculoskeletal neuromuscular impairment from fracture, trauma, falls or abuse
Defining characteristics: Inability to purposefully move within physical environment, impaired gait and coordination, decreased muscle strength, foot problems, loss of physical function, pain and swelling at fracture site

Risk for trauma (198)

Related to: Weakness, lack of safety precautions, cognitive or emotional difficulties, history of previous trauma from neglect, impaired physical/mental condition
Defining characteristics: Bruising of tissue, fracture of bones, unsafe environment, improper medication administration, falls, impaired mobility

SPECIFIC DIAGNOSES AND CARE PLANS

Pain

Related to: Biological injuring agents (fracture, trauma)
Defining characteristics: Communication of pain descriptors, guarding behavior, swelling, tissue bruising

Outcome Criteria

Relief of pain.

Interventions	Rationales
Assess for pain, severity, site, presence of fracture from fall or abuse	Provides information for analgesic administration from pain caused by spasms, edema
Administer analgesic based on pain assessment	Provides relief of pain by effect on CNS pathways
Handle gently when moving or positioning; maintain body alignment	Prevents increased pain with movement
Support injured area with pillows; immobilize part as appropriate	Promotes comfort while immobilized
Maintain traction force if present; unobstructed pulleys	Immobilizes part while healing and decreases pain
Apply ice pack judiciously if appropriate and tactile perception is intact	Reduces swelling and pain

Information, Instruction, Demonstration

Interventions	Rationales
Inform of pain relieving techniques (relaxation, imagery)	Reduces pain

Discharge or Maintenance Evaluation

- Pain relieved or controlled
- Use of nonpharmacological methods to control pain

Post-trauma response

Related to: Assault or neglect (physical abuse)
Defining characteristics: Excessive fear, dependent behavior, avoidance of abuser's touch, blames self, unexplained bruises or fractures, lack of supervision, unsafe environment

Outcome Criteria

Identification, exposure and resolution of abuse against client. Absence of injury, behaviors associated with abuse.

Interventions	Rationales
Assess history of injury, crises and evidence of abuse or neglect, ability to express that abuse has occurred, anger or guilt	Identifies presence of abuse pattern
Assess activities, perceptions regarding injury, cognitive and emotional status	Separates real from imagined causes of injuries
Provide protection from abuser	Prevents continuing abuse
Refer to community legal support and protective services and report if abuse is suspected	Protects client from further abuse or neglect
Provide privacy during assessments and care	Reduces fear, promotes trusting relationship

Information, Instruction, Demonstration

Interventions	Rationales
Inform family about client's physical status	Assists to deal with feelings and maintain contact with client if appropriate

Interventions	Rationales
Inform of actions that provide safe environment, need for supervision	Prevents injury as result of neglect in removing hazards from environment
Suggest counseling for client and/or abuser	Provides support for change in behavior and coping ability

Discharge or Maintenance Evaluation

- Termination of physical abuse or neglect
- Absence of injury, trauma
- Reduction in behaviors associated with past abuse

Risk for injury

Related to: Internal biochemical factors - Sensory dysfunction, integrative dysfunction
Defining characteristics: Change in mentation, alteration in visual, tactile perception, reduction in functional ability of systems and effect of interrelationship of systems, depression

Related to: Internal developmental factors — Aging, decreased cardiac output and cerebral flow, mobility impairment
Defining characteristics: Change in mentation, bone loss, weak muscle, support system, muscle tone, poor posture

Related to: External chemical factors — Pharmaceutical agents
Defining characteristics: Confusion, drowsiness, impaired judgment

Outcome Criteria

No trauma or fracture from falls.

Interventions	Rationales
Assess type of medications, effect of medications, number of medications being taken	Several medications may be prescribed for more than one medical condition; drug absorption, distribution and excretion are altered in the aged causing confusion, forgetfulness leading to falls
Assess accident proneness, presence of agitation, chairbound or ambulatory, interference with thinking, balance, gait, hostility, depression or suicidal tendency, need for attention	Conditions that predispose to falls in the elderly
Maintain vigilance and supervision when needed	Accident prevention maintains safety of client
Reduce unsafe activities and behaviors or modify if appropriate	Reduces risk of falls

Information, Instruction, Demonstration

Interventions	Rationales
Instruct in safe operation of wheelchair, other assistive devices	Promotes safety
Instruct in responsible administration of all medications	Prevents mistakes causing overdoses and untoward side effects leading to accidents

Discharge or Maintenance Evaluation

- No accidental falls
- Absence of fractures or tissue trauma
- Correct administration of medications with use of special aids to assist in memory, reading labels, preparation, written instructions and schedules

Osteoporosis

Aging process

↓   ↓   ↓

Immobility and decreased   Gonad deficiency   Decreased intestinal
weight bearing   Menopause   absorption of Ca

↓   ↓   ↓

Acceleration of bone resorption

↓

Decreased organic matrix and mineral content of bone

↓

Cancellous bone
Thinning of bone cortex

↓

Brittle, fragile bones
Loss of height
Increased kyphosis of dorsal spine
Bone that fractures easily

↓

Pain
Deformity
Spontaneous fracture (mostly hip and vertebrae)

Osteoporosis

Loss of bone mass is common to all elderly and leads to spontaneous or slight trauma fractures. Osteoporosis is bone demineralization caused by mineral resorption that exceeds bone formation resulting in brittle, porous, thinning bones. This occurs in the presence of immobility, decreased estrogen secretion in menopausal women and changes in intestinal absorption of calcium in the elderly. The disorder develops over long periods of time and causes eventual loss in height, kyphosis (widow's hump), shorter trunk and decreased thorax movement leading to respiratory problems and self-image disturbance. Mobility, movement restrictions and tendency for fractures are further complications of a compromised musculoskeletal system.

MEDICAL CARE

Calcium: calcium carbonate (Caltrate, Os-Cal) PO for calcium replacement if intake inadequate

Hormone: estrogen (Premarin) PO in menopausal women to maintain bone mass and retard osteoporosis

Vitamin D: calcifediol (Calderol) PO to regulate serum calcium in management of metabolic bone disease as it is necessary for calcium absorption in the intestines

Sodium fluoride: Adjunct treatment in combination with calcium and vitamin D

X-ray: Reveals bone fracture and degeneration

CT scan: Reveals bone loss

Dual-proton absorptiometry: Reveals bone density

Alkaline phosphatase: Reveals increases in presence of fracture

Serum calcium, phosphorus: Reveals normal levels or slight increases in bone destruction

NURSING CARE PLANS

Essential nursing diagnoses and plans associated with this condition:

Impaired physical mobility (196)

Related to: Pain, discomfort and neuromuscular impairment from bone loss, fracture
Defining characteristics: Inability to move safely within physical environment, reluctance to attempt movement, pain of fracture, presence of fracture restricting movement

Risk for trauma (198)

Related to: Internal factors of bone loss and weakness from bone demineralization causing falls
Defining characteristics: Spontaneous fracture, difficulty bending or climbing stairs, fracture resulting from minimal trauma, unsafe environment, past fractures from falls

SPECIFIC DIAGNOSES AND CARE PLANS

Knowledge deficit

Related to: Lack of exposure to information regarding medications, dietary modifications, safe activity program
Defining characteristics: Verbalization of the problem, request for information, fear of further bone loss and fracture

Outcome Criteria

Increased knowledge and compliance with medical regimen to minimize bone demineralization and injury.

Interventions	Rationales
Assess knowledge of disease and dietary, medication and exercise program to arrest progression of bone deterioration	Provides basis for teaching and techniques to promote compliance; disease not usually detected until 25-40% of calcium in bone is lost
Instruct in methods to perform ADLs and avoid lifting, bending or carrying objects	Prevents injury that can occur with minimal trauma
Assist to plan exercise program according to capabilities; to avoid flexion of spine and wear corset if appropriate (walking is preferred to jogging)	Exercise will strengthen bone; vertebral collapse is common and corset provides support
Instruct in administration of calcium, estrogen therapy, vitamin D	Provides calcium replacement and absorption to arrest bone loss
Assist to plan diet containing calcium (dairy products, green vegetables, fish)	Provides calcium supplement to dietary intake (1000-1500 mg day needed by women)
Refer to physical or occupational therapist if appropriate	Provides exercise and activity program to maintain bone condition and encourage independence in ADL
Provide support of body image and lifestyle changes	Assist client to cope with chronicity of disease and potential fractures causing pain and immobility
Inform of assistive devices and safety precautions available to maintain mobility	Prevents trauma or fracture from falls

Discharge or Maintenance Evaluation

- Compliance with medication and dietary instruction
- Daily exercises within identified limitations
- Absence of injury/fracture from falls
- Independence in performing ADL with environmental modifications

Hip Fracture/Total Hip Replacement

Aging

↓

Altered sensory perception	Osteoporosis Arthritis	Bone cancer or metastasis to bone	Environmental hazard
↓	↓	↓	↓
Reduced or poor vision	Degneration of joint Reduced bone density	Excessive stress on joints	Wet floor Poor lighting Pathway clutter Unsafe use of aids
↓	↓	↓	↓

Falls
Trauma

↓

Fracture

↓

Open reduction of fracture
Total joint replacement

Hip Fracture/ Total Hip Replacement

Fracture of the hip is a common injury of the elderly caused by falls, cancer of the bone, osteoporosis, or excessive stress on the joint. Osteoarthritis is a common joint disease of the elderly. Either can result in corrective surgery such as an open reduction of a fracture or total hip or knee replacement procedure. Open reduction for hip fracture (femoral neck, introtrochanteric) are performed by surgery with the use of pins, nails, compression screw as well as the total replacement or hemiarthroplasty. Total hip replacement is the surgical removal of the ball (femoral head) and socket (acetabulum) of the hip joint and the placement of a prosthetic appliance. Total knee replacement if the surgical removal of the surfaces where the tibia and femur articulate at the knee joint, and of the patella if necessary, with the placement of a prosthesis.

MEDICAL CARE

Analgesics: acetaminophen (Tylenol), ibuprofen (Motrin), oxycodone (Percodan) PO depending on severity of pain

X-ray of joints: Reveals fracture site and type of fracture

Surgery: Joint replacement, pins, nails, or screws for internal reduction of fracture

NURSING CARE PLANS

Essential nursing diagnoses and plans associated with these conditions:

Impaired physical mobility (196)

Related to: Musculoskeletal impairment, intolerance to activity
Defining characteristics: Reluntance to attempt movement, inability to effectively move within physical environment including bed mobility, ambulation, and transfer, fear of falling or dislocating prosthesis, impaired weight bearing and movement of operative side

Risk for trauma (198)

Related to: Internal factor of weakness caused by surgical procedure, external factor of environmental safety hazards
Defining characteristics: Slippery floors, littered pathways, unanchored rugs, poor lighting, unsteady gait or incoordination, improper use of assistive aids for support when ambulating, poor fitting shoes and socks, impaired vision, confusion

SPECIFIC DIAGNOSES AND CARE PLANS

Pain

Related to: Physical injuring agent of trauma from surgical repair or joint replacement
Defining characteristics: Spasms and inflammation following corrective surgery

Outcome Criteria

Pain relieved or controlled

Interventions	Rationales
Assess for pain descriptors, severity, (hip, knee), muscle spasms, edema at site	Provides data regarding need for analgesia
Operative limb and factors that contribute to pain (anxiety, improper positioning of operative side, prolonged immobilization)	Indicates tolerance for pain and activities that increase discomfort
Administer analgesic based on pain assessment	Acts to reduce pain by interfering with CNS pathways
Place extremity in abducted position by suspension or pillows between legs (hip surgery), extremity in proper alignment without flexion beyond recommended degree (knee surgery)	Relieves pain by correct positioning of affect side
Position and move extremity with gentle smooth movements and support	Prevents spasms or pressure that causes pain

Information, Instruction, Demonstration

Interventions	Rationales
Instruct in pain relieving techniques and diversions (relaxation, imagery, music)	Reduces pain

Discharge or Maintenance Evaluation

- Pain relieved
- Uses nonpharmacological methods to increase comfort

Ineffective individual coping

Related to: Multiple lifestyle changes (limitations imposed by injury/surgery)
Defining characteristics: Inability to meet expectations for self-care, chronic fatigue and anxiety, alteration in societal participation

Outcome Criteria

Adaptation to limitations with optimal adjustment in lifestyle in relation to use of extremities for ambulation, and maintenance and participation in ADL

Interventions	Rationales
Assess use of coping skills, ability to cope with lifestyle limitations and changes in activity pattern	Older adults display outstanding ability to cope and adapt, although inability to maintain independence and control over life leads to frustration and negative feelings about lifestyle
Assist to identify positive defense mechanism and promote behaviors to be learned	Use of defense mechanisms that have worked in the past increases ability to cope and promote self-esteem
Provide environment that allows for free expression of concerns and fears	Encourages trust and relieves anxiety
Assess ability to perform daily self-care routines and activities, attitude about accepting assistance if needed	Assists to determine need for assistance or assistive aids to encourage independence and and control over the environment

Information, Instruction, Demonstration

Interventions	Rationales
Social and coping skills with problem-solving approaches	Prevents disengagement and promotes coping with lifestyle changes
Ways or methods to adapt roles to new situation or need	Provides alternatives that increase participation and independence in activities
Suggest support group or therapy if appropriate	Provides a variety of techniques to reduce anxiety and stress

Discharge or Maintenance Evaluation

- Uses appropriate coping and problem-solving skills in adapting to functional changes
- Level of independence appropriate for functional ability
- Requests assistance when needed
- Participates in social activities according to preference and activity tolerance

Knowledge deficit

Related to: Lack of information regarding preservation of independence, mobility and exercises, and rehabilitation regimens

Defining characteristics: Request for information, fear of joint damage during rehabilitation regimen

Outcome Criteria

Adequate knowledge to comply with follow-up care and progressive resumption of routine activities

Interventions	Rationales
Assess knowledge of exercise program according to capabilities, reason for rehabilitation regimen	Provides basis for teaching and techniques to promote compliance
Continue physical therapy and transfer techniques to chair or commode, use of aids for ambulation and personal care (raised toilet seat, walker, cane)	Provides for support and continued rehabilitative progress, independence in self-care
Continue muscle and joint exercises including ROM following rehabilitation regimen	Maintains muscle strength and promotes endurance
Crutch walking, use of walker or cane as appropriate, gait training, weight bearing, use of proper shoes	Allows for mobility, can be non-weight-bearing, partial- or full-weight bearing
Avoid leaning forward, reaching for articles on floor, use of pillow under knees, avoid any extremes related to internal rotation, flexion, or adduction of hip, use long-handled aid for putting on shoes and hose	Prevent hip or knee flexion of more than 90 degrees that can dislocate the prosthesis
Avoid crossing legs, keep the knees parted, lifting heavy objects, prolonged sitting, sitting in low chairs with soft seats	Prevents strain on affected side and possible injury
Avoid position during intercourse that causes hip to turn inward or any rotation of the knee, begin climbing stairs as advised by physician	Prevents positioning that can cause injury or displacement of prosthesis
Keep scheduled appointments for follow-up care, x-rays, rehabilitation therapy as scheduled	Length of time for rehabilitation can continue until ability to ambulate and perform other activities is regained

Discharge or Maintenance Evaluation

- Complies with rehabilitation regimen
- Daily activities within identified limitations
- Modifies environment to enhance independence in exercise/activity program

Hematologic System

Hematologic System

Alterations in the hematologic and immune systems resulting from the aging process revolve around the body's ability to protect itself from infection and neoplastic disorders. There is a definite relationship between a decline in the efficiency of the immune system and an increased vulnerability to cancer as a reduction in the capacity for the immune system to destroy potentially tumor-inducing cell changes allows the aberrant cells to grow. Leukemia, multiple myeloma and lymphosarcoma are the most common neoplasms in the elderly associated with the blood forming organs.

GENERAL HEMATOLOGIC CHANGES ASSOCIATED WITH THE AGING PROCESS

Structural changes

- Atrophy of lymphoid tissue causing decreased immunity
- Gradual degeneration of thymus gland with increased diversification of cells

Functional changes

- Decrease in capacity of bone marrow to produce leukocytes and erythrocytes causing poor response to infection and anemia
- Decrease in antibodies causing a reduced antibody response to antigens
- Reduction or absence of thymic hormone secretion causing a decreased response to antigenic stimuli
- Increase in auto-antibodies causing susceptibility to autoimmune diseases
- Decreased immunocompetence causing reduced potential for survival from disease
- Decreased production and efficiency of T-lymphocytes by thymus causing a reduced ability to respond to antigens and prevent tumor formation

Anemia

Decreased iron intake   Absence of intrinsic factor
↓   ↓

Decrease in hemoglobin synthesis   Lack of binding to
↓ B_{12} when ingested
↓

Decrease in red cells
Decrease in serum iron   Abnormally large RBC with
↓   short life span
Failure of nuclear maturation
causing RBC cell division

Impaired oxygen transport   ←
↓

Tachycardia, palipitations
Dyspnea
Dizziness, fatigue
Pallor

Anemia

Anemia is a decrease in the number of circulating erythrocytes (RBCs), the quantity of hemoglobin (Hgb) and the volume of packed erythrocytes (Hct). In the elderly, it is most commonly caused by inadequate intake of iron in the diet (iron-deficiency anemia), reduction or absence of secretion of a protein known as intrinsic factor by the gastric muscosa needed to absorb vitamin B$_{12}$ (pernicious anemia). Anemia may also develop in the presence of chronic disorders common in the elderly such as chronic renal failure, hypothyroidism, malignancies and hypertension as well as eating disorders precipitated by anorexia, denture, teeth or oral problems, depression, isolation and cognitive deficits.

MEDICAL CARE

Iron supplements: ferrous sulfate (Feosol) PO, iron dextran (Imferon) IM to replace iron in iron-deficiency anemia

Vitamins: cyanocobalamin (B$_{12}$) IM to provide deficient vitamin in pernicious anemia

Transfusions: Whole blood or packed red cells IV to replace blood or RBCs

RBC and RBC indices: Reveals decreased RBC count, MCH decreased, MCV and MCHC decreased in iron deficiency and increased in pernicious anemia

Hemoglobin (Hb): Reveals decreases in anemia

Hematocrit (Hct): Reveals decreases in anemia

Reticulocytes: Reveals decreases in iron-deficiency and pernicious anemia

Iron: Reveals decreases in anemia

Total iron binding capicity (TIBC): Reveals decreases in anemia

Platelets: Reveals increases in iron-deficiency and decreases in pernicious anemia

Schilling test: Reveals positive results in determining amounts of B$_{12}$ excreted in urine to diagnosis pernicious anemia

Ferritin: Reveals decreases in iron-deficiency anemia

Blood typing and cross-matching: Prepares for compatable transfusion

NURSING CARE PLANS

Essential nursing diagnoses and plans associated with this condition:

Altered tissue perfusion: cerebral, cardiopulmonary, renal, gastrointestinal, peripheral (6)

Related to: Exchange problems from reduced oxygenation (hypoxia) caused by reduced RBCs, Hb, Hct
Defining characteristics: Pallor, confusion, dizziness, faintness, dyspnea, BP and P changes, nausea, palpitations

Risk for impaired skin integrity (246)

Related to: Internal factors of altered circulation and metabolic state from nutritional deficiency and hypoxia
Defining characteristics: Irritation or disruption of skin surfaces

Altered nutrition: less than body requirements (118)

Related to: Inability to ingest, digest and absorb nutrients from reduced carrying capacity of nutrients, inability to absorb B_{12}
Defining characteristics: Nausea, anorexia, deficient intake of iron-containing foods, weight loss, sore buccal cavity

SPECIFIC DIAGNOSES AND CARE PLANS

Activity intolerance

Related to: Generalized weakness (fatigue)
Defining characteristics: Verbal report of fatigue and weakness

Related to: Imbalance between oxygen supply and demand (reduced oxygen carrying capacity of blood causing hypoxia)
Defining characteristics: Abnormal heart rate response to activity, exertional discomfort or dyspnea

Outcome Criteria

Endurance and energy necessary to carry out ADL.

Interventions	Rationales
Assess for baseline tolerance for activity, ability to adapt, amount of rest and sleep, weakness, dyspnea	Promotes and protects respiratory function in presence of tissue hypoxia
Assess pulse and respirations before, during and after activity	Pulse increase of 10 or more beats, or an increase and any difficulty in respirations indicate that activity limit has been reached

Interventions	Rationales
Provide periods of rest after activity; schedule activities around rest or sleep periods; allow self-pacing of activities	Prevents dyspneic episode and provides uninterrupted rest and sleep necessary for physical and mental health to prevent fatigue
Assist with care when needed	Conserves energy and reduces demand for oxygen
Provide slow increases in activity and self-care	Builds gradual tolerance to activities and endurance
Provide quiet, stress-free environment	Promotes rest and relaxation to increase endurance and reduce energy demands

Information, Instruction, Demonstration

Interventions	Rationales
Inform client to avoid extending activities beyond fatigue level or tolerance	Prevents fatigue and increased heart rate

Discharge or Maintenance Evaluation

- Activity tolerance within baseline determinations
- Return to respiratory pattern and absence of hypoxia during activities
- Increases endurance and energy during self-care activities

Altered protection

Related to: Abnormal blood profile (anemia)
Defining characteristics: Tissue hypoxia, weakness, malnutrition (iron intake), inability to produce intrinsic factor

Outcome Criteria

Reduced potential for hypoxia, infection.

Interventions	Rationales
Assess presence of activity intolerance, fatigue, weakness	Result of anemia
Administer whole blood or packed red cells as ordered	Replaces needed RBCs to carry oxygen to the cells
Administer iron preparation or vitamin B_{12} IM	Iron replacement treats iron-deficiency and B_{12} pernicious anemia
Offer diet with high iron/folic acid content, high against iron-deficiency as protein inclusions	Provides protection iron is necessary for hemoglobin synthesis

Information, Instruction, Demonstration

Interventions	Rationales
Inform to comply with B_{12} injections and that these must be continued monthly throughout life	Treatment for pernicious anemia
Inform to eat meals that include green, leafy vegetables, eggs, dried fruits, meat, legumes, whole grains	Foods rich in iron content to supply body need to prevent recurrence of anemia; 1 mg iron is absorbed from 10-20 mg of iron ingested with a 5-10% actually absorbed

Discharge or Maintenance Evaluation

- Nutritional iron intake maintained
- Compliance with prescribed B_{12} injections
- RBCs, Hb, Hct within baseline levels for age and sex

Leukemia

Genetic factor   Acquired disease   Chemical and physical agents
↓   ↓   ↓

Transformation of lymphocytes or granulocytes

↓   ↓

Chronic lymphocytic leukemia   Chronic granulocytic leukemia
↓   ↓

Abnormal mature WBC in peripheral circulation
Diffuse replacement of bone marrow with leukemic cells

↓

Infiltration of liver, spleen, lymph nodes and other body tissues
Infection in any organ

↓

Fever, chills, night sweats
Weakness, fatigue (anemia)
Bleeding of skin and mucous membranes (thrombocytopenia)
Weight loss (hypermetabolism of leukemic cells)
Headache, visual disturbances (CNS involvement)
Abdominal tenderness and fullness (hepatomegaly, splenomegaly, lymphadomegaly)

Endocrine System

Endocrine System

Aging influences on the endocrine system are associated with central endocrine deficiencies causing a reduced ability of the body to maintain homokinesis. Disorders and conditions caused by changes in structure and function of the ductless glands in the elderly are the result of an over or under production of hormones and are chronic in nature. Endocrine function is normal at rest but easily becomes dysfunctional under stress.

GENERAL ENDOCRINE CHANGES ASSOCIATED WITH THE AGING PROCESS

Gland structure

- Fibrosis and follicular distended thyroid gland causing no effect in the functioning of the gland
- Some atrophy of the parathyroid gland causing some degree of degeneration of the gland
- Increased amount of connective tissue with a decrease in vascularity of the pituitary gland
- Alveolar degeneration and obstruction of the ducts in the pancreas causing blockage and back pressure as secretion release continues

Physiologic function

- Decreased secretion of triiodothyronine (T_3) by thyroid gland causing decreased metabolic rate
- Increased follicle-stimulating hormone (FSH) by pituitary gland in menopausal state
- Decreased insulin release but increased insulin release when carbohydrate intake is increased causing prolonged hypoglycemia
- Glucose tolerance deterioration causing potential for diabetes mellitus II
- Reduced number of insulin receptors on cells; reduced amount of insulin secreted causing diabetes mellitus II
- Decreased cortisol secretion by adrenal glands with a decrease in excretion rate by the kidneys
- Decreased aldosterone excretion rate and concentration in blood
- Decreased excretion of adrenal androgens (ketosteroids)
- Cessation of estrogen at menopause causing atrophy of uterus, vagina, ovaries
- Decreased anabolic steroid production by gonads causing muscle protein loss
- Decreased progesterone production by ovaries, adrenal gland and testes
- Decreased testosterone production and excretion in males affecting genital tissue in men, causing a gradual decline in sexual energy level and muscle strength; continued production of testosterone in menopausal women

Diabetes Mellitus

Aging, obesity, genetic factors   Viral infections

↓   ↓

NIDDM   IDDM

↓   ↓

Insulin ineffectiveness   Insulin deficiency
Lack of availability

↓   ↓

Glucose remains in plasma and not transferred into cells

↓   ↓

Plasma osmolality increases   Glucose not metabolized for use
by body to supply energy

↓   ↓   ↓

Osmotic diuresis   Hyperglycemia   Breakdown of
fats for energy

↓   ↓   ↓

Polyuria   Glycosuria   Ketoacidosis
Polydipsia   Ketouria
Polyphagia

Diabetes Mellitus

Diabetes mellitus is a chronic disorder affecting the elderly characterized by absence of, insufficient secretion of, or ineffective utilization of insulin. It is classified as Type I (IDDM) or insulin dependent or Type II (NIDDM) or non-insulin dependent. The disease causes impaired metabolism of carbohydrates, proteins, and fats.

MEDICAL CARE

Oral hypoglycemics (sulfonylureas): glipizide (Glucotrol), glyburide (Micronase), PO to stimulate beta cells to release insulin in NIDDM

Insulin: Immediate acting (Regular), intermediate-acting (NPH), long-acting (Ultralente) SC given individually or in combination to provide insulin replacement

Blood glucose: Fasting sample reveals circulating glucose level of 140 mg/dL or more which indicates potential for diabetes; two hour postprandial sample reveals 180 mg/dL or more in presence of diabetes

Glucose tolerance: Reveals two or more increases of 200 mg/dL after glucose ingestion

Capillary glucose: Reveals glucose level by Chemstrip and glucometer

Urinary analysis: Reveals glycosuria as blood levels reach 180 mg/dL tested for glucose and ketones by Ketodiastix

Glycosyiated hemoglobin: Reveals glucose and hemoglobin linkage to determine effectiveness of glucose control

NURSING CARE PLANS

Essential nursing diagnoses and plans associated with this condition:

Altered tissue perfusion: cerebral, cardiopulmonary, gastrointestinal, renal, peripheral (6)

Related to: Interruption of arterial flow from macro/microangiopathies and atherosclerosis
Defining characteristics: Vasoconstriction, hypotension with increased pulse and respirations; mental cloudiness, carotid bruits, oliguria, retinopathy, nephropathy, dermopathy, intermittent claudication, cold feet, hair loss, dependent rubor, delayed capillary filling, gangrene

Sensory/perceptual alteration: visual, tactile (72)

Related to: Altered sensory reception, transmission and/or integration of neurological deficit from neuropathy or altered status of sense organ from retinopathy
Defining characteristics: Decreased visual acuity, glaucoma, cataract formation; pain and paresthesias of extremities, tingling, burning, itching sensations, loss of sensitivity to touch and temperature changes with feeling of numbness

Sexual dysfunction (181)

Related to: Altered body function of disease process from neuropathy affecting autonomic nervous system
Defining characteristics: Impotence, inability to achieve desired satisfaction, verbalization of the problem

Risk for trauma (198)

Related to: Internal factors — Reduced temperature and tactile sensation and ankle and foot changes from neuropathic arthropathy and impaired sensory perception neuropathy
Defining characteristics: Joint dysfunction, foot drop, ulceration of leg or foot, burns or bruising of - legs, slow healing and necrosis of leg ulcer

Risk for impaired skin integrity (246)

Related to: Internal factors of altered circulation, altered pigmentation from microangiopathy
Defining characteristics: Brown spots on lower extremities, ulceration and necrosis of skin on legs, reduced tactile sensitivity in legs

Functional incontinence (154)

Related to: Neuropathy affecting the autonomic nervous system
Defining characteristics: Decreased awareness of bladder fullness, urinary retention, infrequent voiding, difficulty voiding, nocturia, incontinence, weak stream of urine

Altered nutrition: more than body requirements (118)

Related to: Excessive intake in relationship to metabolic need causing obesity and decreasing insulin receptors in skeletal muscle and fat cells (peripheral insulin resistance)
Defining characteristics: Weight 10% or more over ideal for height and frame, dysfunctional eating pattern, lack of control of hyperglycemia

SPECIFIC DIAGNOSES AND CARE PLANS

Risk for infection

Related to: Chronic disease with glycosuria, impaired phagocytosis of WBCs
Defining characteristics: Urinary infection. vaginitis, skin infections

Outcome Criteria

Absence of infectious process with glucose levels within baseline determinations.

Interventions	Rationales
Assess urine for cloudiness and foul odor, sediment	Indicates urinary infection resulting from glycosuria
Assess for vaginal itching, burning, foul-smelling discharge; skin eruptions or infections containing pus	Indicates vaginitis, boil or furucle formation caused by failure to immobilize inflammatory cells and ineffective WBC activity
Administer anti-infectives (antibiotics or antifungals) PO or via vaginal suppository	Prevents or treats bacterial or fungal (*Candida*) infections
Maintain daily bathing and foot care schedule	Promotes cleanliness and prevents breaks in skin of feet; poor circulation and risk for infection causes difficulty in healing
Clean perineal area after each voiding, bowel elimination; wipe from front to back in female	Prevents bacterial contamination of meatal orifice

Information Instruction, Demonstration

Interventions	Rationales
Cleansing of perineal area; use commercial wipes if appropriate	Removes remaining contaminants after elimination
Instruct to wash feet daily with mild soap, tepid water, pat dry carefully between toes as well as feet; report irritations or breaks in skin or reduced sensation	Prevents infection
Suggest changing socks daily, cotton preferred, avoiding tight socks or large socks that cause shoes to fit tightly	Maintains cleanliness, dryness and avoids pressure to feet
Suggest use of light powder, soft padding between toes	Maintains dryness and relieves pressure
Inform to change shoes every day, to wear good fitting, comfortable shoes	Prevents pressure on skin
Suggest podiatrist for cutting toenails, trimming corns or calluses	Prevents nicking skin when trimming nails
Instruct to carry out mouth care twice a day	Prevents oral fungal infection

Discharge or Maintenance Evaluation

- No evidence of infection of skin or mucous membranes
- Feet clean and skin intact with compliance of foot care
- Verbalizes causes of infection and steps to take to prevent potential for infection

Knowledge deficit

Related to: Lack of information about disease process and care (medication, dietary and exercise regimen, testing for glucose level)
Defining characteristics: Verbalization of the problem, request for information, new diagnosis of NIDDM, coversion from NIDDM to IDDM

Outcome Criteria

Appropriate knowledge of medical regimen prescribed to control hyperglycemia/hypoglycemia.

Interventions	Rationales
Assess knowledge of factors associated with disease and methods to control and stabilize diabetes	Prevents repetition of information and promotes compliance necessary to maintain normal glucose level
Provide information and explanations in clear, simple language that is understandable; provide limited amounts of information over time	Encourages compliance of medical regimen according to cognitive ability and readiness
Use pictures, pamphlets, video tapes, models in teaching	Provides visual aids to reinforce learning
Inform of possible symptoms to report including nausea, drowsiness, lethargy, polyuria, blood glucose of 240 mg/dL or more	May lead to diabetic hyperglycemic coma
Inform of possible hypoglycemia symptoms to report including shaky feeling, nervousness, confusion, hunger, weakness and to take orange juice, honey or sugar to counteract this reaction	May lead to insulin shock

Interventions	Rationales
Instruct client to take oral hypoglycemic daily before breakfast or meals in divided doses; name, action and side effects of medication	Promotes correct dosage at correct times to control NIDDM
Instruct in administration of insulin; name, action, peak levels, dosage, how to store, preparation and filling syringe, rotation of sites and procedure to inject insulin	Ensures correct dosage to control IDDM, if able to administer own insulin
Instruct and assist to develop menus for appropriate caloric and food selections using American Diabetic Association guidelines provide sample menus and exchange lists	Dietary management controls NIDDM and is also necessary to adjust insulin dosage
Instruct not to skip meals, avoid fad diets, high sugar and carbohydrate desserts, alcohol	Food intake is calculated to correlate with insulin and exercise program; alcohol inhibits gluconeogenesis
Instruct in blood and urine testing using Ketostix or Testape, Chemstrip and Glucometer analysis of capillary blood; obtaining samples of blood and urine	Provides glucose levels in blood and urine to determine presence of hypo- or hyperglycemia, glycosuria and ketones
Provide daily exercise/activity program; to avoid overactivity or strenuous activities, use of a carbohydrate if activity is increased	Activity is essential for optimal results of medical regimen by utilization of diet and medication

Discharge or Maintenance Evaluation

- Statements of knowledge of disease, medications, diet and exercise requirements
- Blood and urine glucose levels within baseline levels
- Adaptation and compliance with medical regimen
- Verbalization of complications of hypo- or hyperglycemia to report
- Plans menus for diabetic diet with proper modifications if needed (sodium or cholesterol restriction) using ADA guidelines
- Appropriate body weight maintained for age, height and frame
- Demonstrates blood and urine collection and testing correctly and maintains log of results

Thyroid Dysfunction

The thyroid conditions most commonly found in the elderly are thyrotoxicosis or increases in circulating thyroid hormones causing an increase in body functions; or hypothyroidism or the decrease or absence of circulating thyroid hormones causing a decrease in body functions. Hormone secretions associated with thyroid function are calcitonin, thyroxine (T_4), triiodothyronine (T_3) from the thyroid gland, thyroid-stimulating hormone (TSH) from the anterior pituitary gland and thyrotropin-releasing hormone (TRH) from the hypothalamus.

MEDICAL CARE

Thyroid hormones: levothyroxine (Synthroid), dessicated thyroid (Armour) PO as thyroid replacement to treat hypothyroidism

Antithyroids: propylthiouracil (Propacil) PO to block synthesis of thyroid hormones to treat hyperthyroidism

Artificial tears: methylcellulose (Tearisol) eye drops for comfort in exophthalmos

Thyroid scan: Reveals thyroid function and nodules

Chest x-ray: Reveals enlarged heart in hypothyroidism

Electrocardiogram: Reveals cardiac abnormalities in the hypo- or hyperthyroidism

Thyroxine (T_4) and triiodothyronine (T_3): Reveals thyroid function when done by radioimmunoassay technique (RIA) of increased levels in hyperthyroidism and decreased levels in hypothyroidism

Triiodothyronine resin uptake (T_3RU): Reveals thyroid binding globulin capacity (TCB) with increases in hyperthyroidism and decreases in hypothyroidism

Radioactive iodine uptake (RAIU): Reveals thyroid activity by measuring time of uptake of a dose of I^{131}

Thyroid-stimulating hormone (TSH): Reveals increases in diagnosis of hypothyroidism

Cholesterol: Reveals increases in hypothyroidism and decreases in hyperthyroidism

Alkaline phosphatase: Reveals increases in hyperthyroidism and hypothyroidism

NURSING CARE PLANS

Essential nursing diagnoses and plans associated with these conditions:

Fluid volume excess (8)

Related to: Compromised regulatory mechanisms from decreased thyroid hormone (hypothyroidism)
Defining characteristics: Interstitial edema, face puffiness, periorbital edema, weight gain.

Decreased cardiac output (4)

Related to: Alterations in inotropic (contractility) changes in heart from decreased thyroid hormone (hypothyroidism)
Defining characteristics: Bradycardia, hypotension, dyspnea, decreased peripheral circulation

Altered thought processes (70)

Related to: Physiological changes from decreased thyroid hormone (hypothyroidism) causing mucoprotein deposits on cranial nerves and diminished blood flow to brain

Thyroid Dysfunction

Aging

↓

Atrophy of thyroid gland
Reduced antithyroid production

↓

Decreased thyroid prodution

↓

Slowing of body processes
Personality changes

↓

Bradycardia, decreased cardiac output
Decreased gastrointestinal motility
Decreased erythropoiesis
Mental sluggishness, lethargy
Dry, coarse skin and hair
Cold intolerance
Decreased metabolism
Decresed musble tone, weakness
Sexual dysfunction, menorrhagia
Weight gain

Increased secretion of thyroid hormones
Diffuse thyroid hyperplasia

↓   ↓

Increase in oxygen con-   Edema of orbital
sumption   structure
Increase in metabolism
Increase in sympathetic   ↓
activity

Graves' disease
→   ←

↓

Weight loss
Tachycardia, increased cardiac output
Irritability, fatigue
Heat intolerance
Diarrhea
Thin, silky skin and hair
Increased muscle tone
Retraction of eyelids

Defining characteristics: Lethargy, apathy, forgetfulness, inattentativeness, decreased intellectual functioning

Risk for impaired skin integrity (246)

Related to: Internal factors of altered metabolic state from decreased thyroid hormone (hypothyroidism) causing mucopolysaccharide deposits in subcutaneous tissues
Defining characteristics: Thick, dry, leathery skin, thick, brittle nails, sparse, coarse hair on head and eyebrows

Constipation (121)

Related to: Gastrointestinal impairment from decreased thyroid hormone (hypothyroid) causing decreased motility
Defining characteristics: Less frequent bowel elimination, hard-formed stool, reported feeling of rectal fullness

Altered nutrition: more than body requirements (120)

Related to: Excessive intake in relationship to metabolic need from decreased thyroid hormone (hypothyroidism) causing reduced metabolic rate
Defining characteristics: Weight gain, poor appetite, low energy

Altered nutrition: less than body requirements (118)

Related to: Biologic factors from increased thyroid hormone (hyperthyroidism) causing increased metabolism
Defining characteristics: Weight loss in spite of appetite and adequate intake, nausea, vomiting

Diarrhea (122)

Related to: Internal factor from increased thyroid hormone (hyperthyroidism) causing increased bowel motility
Defining characteristics: Increased bowel sounds, frequent loose stools, abdominal cramping

Sleep pattern disturbance (77)

Related to: Internal factor of illness from increased thyroid hormone (hyperthyroidism) causing increased CNS activity
Defining characteristics: Insomnia, restlessness, nervousness, irritability, tremor, interrupted sleep

Sexual dysfunction (181)

Related to: Altered body function from increased or decreased thyroid hormone (hyperthyroidism or hypothyroidism) causing changes in secretions of androgens and progesterone
Defining characteristics: Impotence, decreased libido, inability to achieve desired satisfaction, amenorrhea, menorrhagia, infertility

SPECIFIC DIAGNOSES AND CARE PLANS

Anxiety

Related to: Change in health status (CNS stimulation from hyperthyroidism)
Defining characteristics: Irritability, agitation, insomnia

Outcome Criteria

Reduced anxiety and responses to manageable level.

Interventions	Rationales
Assess sleep pattern, expressions of uncertainty, loss of control, anxiety	Increased CNS stimulation by oversecretion of thyroid creates potential for anxiety
Avoid exposure to stressful situations, confrontation or extra stimulation	May trigger increased anxiety and personality changes
Provide quiet, calm environment	Prevents anxiety caused by stimulation

Information, Instruction, Demonstration

Interventions	Rationales
Inform that irritability, anxiety will decrease when condition is treated and thyroid secretion decreased	Knowledge will reduce anxiety

Discharge or Maintenance Evaluation

- Anxiety relieved or decreased
- Verbalizes reasons for behavior changes and increased anxiety level

Hyperthermia

Related to: Increased metabolic rate (hyperthyroidism)
Defining characteristics: Diaphoresis, heat intolerance

Outcome Criteria

Increased comfort in environmental temperature.

Interventions	Rationales
Assess for perceptions of hot environment, diaphoresis	Impaired temperature adaptation caused by increased secretion of thyroid hormones
Provide well-ventilated room that is cool	Prevents actual or perceived hot feeling
Provide frequent bathing or sponging, change of linen if diaphoretic	Promotes comfort

Information, Instruction, Demonstration

Interventions	Rationales
Suggest cool, loose-fitting clothing that is lightweight	Prevents hot feeling
Inform to drink at least 2 L/day of fluid if diaphoretic	Prevents dehydration from fluid loss

Discharge or Maintenance Evaluation

- Verbalized comfort in environmental temperature
- Absence of diaphoresis, temperature elevation

Risk for injury

Related to: Internal biochemical factor of sensory dysfunction (exophthalmos)
Defining characteristics: Decreased blinking, inability to close eyes, irritation to eyes

Outcome Criteria

Absence of injury to eyes.

Interventions	Rationales
Assess visual acuity, sclera for clearness, cornea for damage, irritation or dryness of eyes	Results from hyperthyroidism with exophthalmos with potential for corneal ulceration
Provide eye pads, tape lids shut if difficult to close	Protects eyes from environmental particles
Provide isotonic eye drops, cool compresses to eyes	Promotes comfort for dry, irritated eyes
Raise head of bed during rest or sleep	Promotes fluid drainage from periorbital area

Information, Instruction, Demonstration

Interventions	Rationales
Suggest sunglasses	Protects eyes from bright lights or particles from environment
Instruct in exercising extraocular muscles	Maintains ocular movement

Discharge or Maintenance Evaluation

- Eyes remain free of irritation or corneal damage
- Compliance in use of eye drops and protective measures for eyes

Fatigue

Related to: Decreased metabolic energy production (hypothyroidism)
Defining characteristics: Verbalization of fatigue/ lack of energy, inability to maintain usual routines, emotionally labile, lethargic

Outcome Criteria

Increased energy and activity tolerance.

Interventions	Rationales
Assess activity tolerance, sleep pattern	Determines baseline for activity limitations to prevent fatigue
Assist to plan schedule of paced activities, rest, exercise within tolerance level	Maintains activity while preventing fatigue
Provide quiet, stress-free environment	Promotes rest and prevents anxiety resulting from increased stimuli

Information, Instruction, Demonstration

Interventions	Rationales
Avoid activities beyond level of tolerance; ask for assistance when needed	Conserves energy
Place articles within reach, use energy-saving devices when possible	Prevents unnecessary activity and fatigue
Importance of rest, nutrition and exercise	Maintains basic needs necessary to prevent fatigue

Discharge or Maintenance Evaluation

- Minimal fatigue level associated with activity limitations
- Statements of interest in activity and fatigue reduction
- Able to participate in activity with performance limited to activity tolerance

Hypothermia

Related to: Decreased metabolic rate (hypothyroidism)
Defining characteristics: Shivering, cool skin, perceived feeling of coldness

Outcome Criteria

Increased comfort in environmental temperature.

Interventions	Rationales
Assess for perception of cold, chilling, shivering	Impaired temperature adaptation caused by decreased secretion of thyroid hormones
Provide warmer clothing, additional blankets, increased environmental temperature	Promotes comfort and warmth

Information, Instruction, Demonstration

Interventions	Rationales
Inform that cold intolerance will decrease with treatment	Information promotes understanding of condition
Suggest warm liquids	Provides warmth

Discharge or Maintenance Evaluation

- Verbalized comfort in environmental temperature with treatment
- Absence of chilling and shivering feeling

Pain

Related to: Biological injury agents (mucinous deposits in joints and muscles from hypothyroidism)
Defining characteristics: Communication of pain descriptors, protective behavior of joints in extremities, hypoactive reflexes, decreased motor activity, muscle strength

Outcome Criteria

Joint and muscle pain relieved or eliminated.

Interventions	Rationales
Assess for pain severity, location, effect on mobility and activity	Effects of decreased thyroid hormone secretion
Handle limbs gently and slowly, use pillow for support	Prevents excessive discomfort
Use bed cradle, padding to extremities	Reduces pressure to limbs that causes pain
Apply splint to joint if appropriate	Provides support to joint

Information, Instruction, Demonstration

Interventions	Rationales
Inform to protect extremities from bumping or weight of clothing	Increases pain
Inform that pain will be controlled with treatment of hormone replacement	Decreases anxiety associated with pain

Discharge or Maintenance Evaluation

- Absence of pain in joints or muscles
- Ability to maintain mobility with compliance in thyroid replacement
- Increased activity tolerance with decreased pain
- Return of muscle tone and strength and coordination with reduced pain

Integumentary System

Integumentary System

In part, the genetic effect on body build and the nutritional status of the elderly determine the amount of fat in the subcutaneous tissue layer. This can mask or accentuate the process and effect of aging on the integumentary system. Because aging changes of the skin and appendages are so visible, they are more traumatic and disturbing to self-esteem and body image. They also predispose to problems with body temperature control, skin breakdown or decubiti, easy bruising and skin discolorations.

GENERAL INTEGUMENTARY CHANGES ASSOCIATED WITH THE AGING PROCESS

Structural changes

- Reduced distribution of body fat; loss of subcutaneous fat especially over the arms and legs causing loss of body insulation and support for vessels
- Reduced formation of collagen with loss of elasticity of skin causing sagging, wrinkles, lines in face and neck, ptosis of eyelids and longation of ear lobes
- Excessive skin pigmentation on exposed areas causing aging spots

- Increased dryness, thinness and vascular fragility of the skin causing increased potential for trauma, itching, bruising
- Skin turgor with decreased water and connective tissue causing stiffness and loss of pliability
- Overgrowth of epidermal tissue causing senile telangiectasia and hyperkeratotic warts
- Increased number and prominence of nail ridges and thickening of toenails with lifting of nail plate causing potential for fungal infections
- Increased thickness, brittleness and splitting of finger nails causing decreased growth and strength as circulation to the area decreases
- Decrease in density of hair follicles causing shining and loss of axillary and pubic hair
- Increased hair growth in ears, nares, eyebrows and hair loss on head (balding) in men

Physiologic function

- Decreased cell replacement in dermis and epidermis causing decreased wound healing and potential for decubiti
- Decreased circulation to skin and appendages causing decreased blood supply of oxygen and nutrients to skin
- Atrophy of skin layers and reduced vascularity and elasticity causing loss of water content and storage in skin layers, reduced turgor, stiffness and loss of pliability
- Decreased water content of skin causing rough, scaly texture and pruritis from dryness and potential for decubiti and trauma
- Neurosensory changes in skin causing absence of tactile perception of pain associated with lesions or growths
- Reduced activity of sebaceous and sweat glands causing dry skin and impaired ability of body to cool itself
- Loss of melanin production causing greying of hair
- Decreased estrogen after menopause causing hair growth on face

ESSENTIAL DIAGNOSES AND CARE PLANS

Risk for impaired skin integrity

Related to: External mechanical factors — Shearing forces, pressure or restraint
Defining characteristics: Bedrest, immobility, reddish-brown color, warmth, firmness of area, corn, - callous formation, disruption of skin surface, pressure from splint or appliance

Related to: External factors — Radiation, physical immobilization, excretions and secretions
Defining characteristics: Reddened, irritated perianal tissue, burning and soreness of perianal skin, irritation, excoriation of skin, maceration of skin

Related to: internal factors — Alteration in nutritional state, altered metabolic state, altered circulation, altered sensation, altered pigmentation, skeletal prominence, alteration in skin turgor (elasticity)
Defining characteristics: Thinning, shiny skin on extremities, brown spots on extremities, irritation of skin areas, thick, dry, leathery skin, brittle nails, jaundice, pruritis, scratching, uric crystals on skin, reduced tactile perception (pressure, pain, heat/cold), dermatitis on skin (food, medication, allergic response)

Outcome Criteria

Skin remains intact and free from irritation and trauma.

Interventions	Rationales
Assess skin, soft tissue especially over bony prominences for color changes, warmth and firmness	Reveals potential for disruption of skin surfaces resulting from pressure, friction or shearing forces
Assess mobility status, ability to move in bed	Immobility is the most common cause of skin impairment

Interventions	Rationales
Assess for skin disruptions, rashes, use of splints, skin growths exposed to pressure	Predisposes to skin breakdown
Assess fecal and urinary continence status, presence of urinary or fecal diversion and peristomal skin condition for excoriation	Dampness and irritation of body secretions and excretion predisposes to skin breakdown
Assess ability to interpret touch by applying hands	Indicates degree of loss of tactile perception
Assess skin dryness, lack of subcutaneous tissue, edema, presence of varicose veins and discoloration of lower extremities	Results of circulatory insufficiency leading to skin breakdown as perfusion of oxygen and nutrients reduced
Apply skin barrier if appropriate, avoid use of tape unless porous type	Protects skin from irritating excretions and materials
Provide position change q2h, maintain body alignment and support with pillows, pads	Unrelieved pressure on skin and soft tissues reduce circulation and predispose to skin breakdown; proper body alignment prevents contractures
Pad bony prominences and susceptible parts without circulation	Promotes circulation and comfort and prevents skin compromising breakdown
Remove splints, antiembolic hose and wash skin daily; apply mild lotion	Prevents irritation of skin under appliance or hose and provides moisture to dry skin
Provide daily foot care by washing and rinsing with mild soap and warm water, dry well and gently including between toes with soft cloth	Prevents infection and protects from ulcer formation

Interventions	Rationales
Place protective pads between toes	Prevents pressure on skin
Provide heat lamp if appropriate	Maintains dryness of irritated area on skin
Maintain wrinkle-free bed, change if wet or soiled	Prevents irritation to skin
Raise head o -bed no higher than semi-Fowler's if tolerated	Elevated head promotes pressure and friction from sliding effect
Provide bath containing oatmeal and sodium bicarbonate as soak and allow to air dry; remove uremic frost with sponge bath as needed	Allays itching in pruritis and promotes comfort

Information, Instruction, Demonstration

Interventions	Rationales
Inform to refrain from scratching skin and apply pressure to area to relieve itching	Prevents breaks in skin from scratches
Inform to test water temperature with thermometer before bath or soak	Maintains temperature no higher than 115°F to prevent burns if sensation reduced
Inform to prevent bumping of extremities on furniture	May cause breaks in fragile, thin skin
Refer to podiatrist for foot care and nail trimming	Prevents accidental nicking or trauma to feet
Avoid going barefoot and exposing feet to extremes of heat and cold	Prevents trauma to feet if circulation or sensation impaired

Interventions	Rationales
Avoid use of commercial products on feet for corns or calluses	Contains harsh chemicals that may injure skin
Inform to maintain mobility and avoid prolonged sitting or lying position	Maintains circulation and prevents pressure on tissues
Inform to use lotions and oils to apply to skin and nails	Prevents skin dryness
Instruct in cleansing of perianal area after each elimination	Cleanses skin and removes excreta that predisposes to skin breakdown

Discharge or Maintenance Evaluation

- Skin free of redness, irritation, burns, bruising, rashes
- Preventative and protective measures taken to prevent skin damage or breakdown
- Compliance with daily skin and foot care
- Effective removal of secretions and excretions from skin
- Skin turgor, moisture, pliability maintained with appropriate fluid intake, lotion application
- Pruritis relieved or controlled

Decubitus Ulcer

Aging

↓   ↓   ↓

Immobility   Decrease in circulation,   Incontinence
nutrients to periphery

↓   ↓   ↓

Restricted movements →   Moisture
Fixed position →   External pressure
Displacement of tissue →   Friction   ↓
Shearing force   Skin macreation

↓   ↓

Disruption of blood flow to   Skin beakdown
capillary beds and arterioles   ↓
Stretching or rupture to
blood vessels   Decubitus ulcer

↓

Edema, autolysis of cells

↓

Tissue ischemia

↓

Decubitus ulcer

Decubitus Ulcer

Decubitus ulcer (pressure sore) is the result of pressure unevenly exerted over any part of the body especially over bony prominences. it occurs whether in seated or supine position when the blood pressure of the skin capillaries is increased enough to interrupt blood flow and cause ischemia. A great amount of pressure over a small area will be more likely to break down than a small amount of pressure applied to a large area. The lesions are graded according to skin damage as follows:

Grade I

Abrasion of the dermis with warm, reddish-brown hard, swollen area

Grade II

Involves all soft tissue with shallow, full thickness ulcer and skin color changes

Grade III

Extension of ulcer to dermis, epidermis and subcutaneous fat with infection and foul odor; open and draining

Grade IV

Large open would involving deep fascia, muscle and bone

MEDICAL CARE

Enzyme debriding agents: fibrinolysin and desoxyribonuclease (Elase), sutilains (Travase) TOP applied to reduce necrotic material

Wound cleansers: dextranomer (Debrisan) TOP to absorb tissue exudate and remove bacteria and protein degradation products; reduces healing time by preventing scab formation and decreasing inflammation and edema

NURSING CARE PLANS

Essential nursing diagnoses and plans associated with this condition

Altered tissue perfusion: peripheral (6)

Related to: Interruption of arterial, venous flow from pressure, friction, shearing force to skin
Defining characteristics: Reddish-brown color to skin, pressure changes, slow healing, tissue edema, impaired tissue nutrition and oxygenation, ulcer formation

Sensory/perceptual alterations: tactile (72)

Related to: Altered status of sense organ from aging process, immobility
Defining characteristics: Reported loss of sensation when pressure applied, posture alteration, inability to change position or feel pain

Functional incontinence (154)

Related to: Sensory, cognitive or mobility deficits
Defining characteristics: Intermittent loss of urine, no awareness of bladder filling or urge to void

SPECIFIC DIAGNOSES AND CARE PLANS

Impaired skin integrity

Related to: External mechanical factors (shearing, pressure, friction), external factor (physical immobilization), internal factors (altered nutritional state, circulation, sensation, skeletal prominence)
Defining characteristics: Disruption of skin surface, skin discoloration, destruction of skin layers

Outcome Criteria

Skin intact with absence of internal or external factors that predispose to skin impairment.

Interventions	Rationales
Assess risk for pressure sore formation with the Norton scale chart or Braden scale	A Norton score of 12-15 indicates a high risk for decubitus formation; apvar or severely limited status level in areas indicates a prediction of risk for decubitus in the Braden scale
Assess skin over bony prominences, soft tissue for reddish-brown color, warmth, firmness, induration, drainage, foul odor	Signs of impending or existence of decubitus ulcer with most common sites at sacrum, heels, elbows, trochanters, scapulae
Assess mobility status, presence of urinary/fecal incontinence, ability to move in bed, sensitivity to pain, edema	Most common causes of decubitus in elderly
Provide position change q2h, maintain body alignment and support with pillows, trochanter rolls, pads	Unrelieved pressure will cause beginning skin breakdown; proper position and support prevents contractures

Interventions	Rationales
Administer debriding or wound cleansing agents as appropriate	Absorbs tissue exudate and assists in healing in stages III and IV decubitus
Wash, rinse and dry skin with mild soap, warm water, soft towel after each incontinent episode; apply skin barrier if appropriate or external devices	Removes body excretions that macerate skin and predispose to breakdown
Maintain bed that is wrinkle and crumb free; change if wet or soiled	Prevents discomfort and ulcer formation
Protect all bony prominences; avoid positioning on any reddish or pink area	Prevents compromised circulation that reduces oxygen and nutrients to tissues
Apply treatments as appropriate (heat lamp, irrigations, wet to dry compresses, whirlpool)	Promotes healing of decubitus
Raise head of bed no higher than semi-Fowler's if tolerated	Elevated head of bed promotes pressure on lower torso from sliding causing friction

Information, Instruction, Demonstration

Interventions	Rationales
Inform of need for fluid intake of at least 2 L/day, high protein dietary intake; suggest nutritionist if appropriate	Promotes tissue integrity and wound healing which is slower in the elderly
Maintain mobility, avoid sitting or lying for prolonged periods	Maintains circulation and prevents pressure on tissues

Interventions	Rationales
Inform how to care for skin and complications of immobility	Promotes knowledge of skin protection

Discharge or Maintenance Evaluation

- Decubitus ulcer formation prevented
- Restoration of skin integrity with appropriate treatment modalities
- Infection and necrosis prevented
- Progressive wound healing process of open decubitus
- Compliance with fluid intake and dietary inclusions of protein and carbohydrate increased

Bunions, Calluses, Corns

Aging

↓ ↓ ↓ ↓

Atrophic, dry, scaling skin	Loss of subcutaneous fat Reduced protective padding	Long-time stressor from weight-bearing and shoes Walking habits Improper fitting shoes	Arthritis contractures, deformities of feet

↓ ↓ ↓ ↓

Pressure on vulnerable area

↓ ↓

Accumulation of or buildup of stratum corneam to protect area from pressure

Elargement of bony prominence on food (large toe joint)

↓ ↓

Formation of callus

Bunion

↓ ↓

Continued pressure
Formation of nucleus in center of callus

Lateral displacement of toe
Thickened bursa of joint

↓

Formation of corn

↓

Pain on pressure of tight shoes
Mobility difficulty

↓

Ulceration
Necrosis

Foot Conditions

Foot pain and disability are common complaints of the elderly. Although causes are classified into mechanical, arthritic, neurotrophic, dermatologic and circulatory, only mechanical and dermatologic disturbances are covered in this plan (the others are covered elsewhere as they relate to respective body systems). Anatomic or pathomechanical changes are responsible for bunions, calluses and corns and deformities such as hallux valgus (displacedtoe) and digitus flexus (hammertoe) all of which place severe limitations on mobility. Dermatological problems common in the elderly include onychocryptosis (ingrown toenail), onychauxis (nail plate thickening) and onychomycosis (fungal infection)

MEDICAL CARE

Keratolytics: urea (Carmol) TOP to soften dry scaly skin by increasing water binding capacity of stratum corneum

Anti-infectives: haloprogin (Halotex) TOP to treat Tinea fungal infection

NURSING CARE PLANS

Essential nursing diagnoses and plans associated with these conditions:

Risk for impaired skin integrity (246)

Related to: External mechanical factor from pressure or trauma

Defining characteristics: Presence of bunion, corn, calluses, nail thickening

Impaired physical mobility (196)

Related to: Musculoskeletal impairment and pain from foot disorder
Defining characteristics: Reluctance to attempt movement, poor-fitting shoes, inflammation, infection, displacement of toe(s), lesion on foot

SPECIFIC DIAGNOSES AND CARE PLANS

Chronic pain

Related to: Chronic physical disability (lesion or impairment of feet)
Defining characteristics: Verbal report of pain for more than 6 months, altered ability to continue previous activities, guarded movements

Outcome Criteria

Foot discomfort relieved.

Interventions	Rationales
Assess feet for pain, lesions, effect on gait, mobility, infection or inflammation of nail, position of toes, presence of spurs or other protrusions on feet	Hyperkerotonic and foot deformities, susceptibility to infections, trauma and poor foot care cause discomfort and affect mobility
Apply pads on corns or calluses and between toes	Reduces pressure that causes pain
Soak toes and/or feet in warm water	Relieves discomfort

Onychauxis, Onychocryptosis, Onychomycosis

Injury to nail
↓

Invasion by *Tinea rubrum* or
mentagrophytes at tip of nails
(fungus)
↓

Digestion of keratin by organisms
↓

Opaque, scaly, hypertrophic nails
Yellow striations
Foul odor
↓

Spread to entire nail
↓

Nail thickening and cracking
Separation from nail bed
↓

Spread to other nails
↓

Onychomycosis

Improper trimming of nail
External pressure
↓

Nail segment penetrates
nail groove as it grows
↓

Pain
Swelling
Redness
Inflammation
↓

Onychocryptosis

Arterosclerosis
Repeated trauma
↓

Nail plate thickening
↓

Onychauxis

Information, Instruction, Demonstration

Interventions	Rationales
Inform client to buy well-fitting shoes that do not pinch or are too tight but stay on well and don't slip	Prevents placing pressure on foot disorder with shoes
Avoid walking barefoot	May increase pain by bumping sore areas on feet

Discharge or Maintenance Evaluation

- Statements that feet are free of pain
- Absence of pain when walking

Risk for infection

Related to: Inadequate primary defenses (broken skin, traumatized tissue

Defining characteristics: Fungal invasion of nail(s), opaque, scaly, hypertrophic nails, foul odor to material under nail, yellow striation of nail, pain, swelling, redness at nail groove, nail thickening and cracking, improperly trimmed nails

Outcome Criteria

Feet and nails free from inflammation and infection.

Interventions	Rationales
Assess toenails and feet for pain, redness, swelling, lifting of nail with material accumulating under it, ability to give nails daily care, injury or trauma to feet	Signs and symptoms of inflammation or infection; improper foot care results in these problems especially if circulatory or sensory deficits present

Interventions	Rationales
Wash feet daily with mild soap and warm water; dry carefully between toes and apply an oil based lotion	Promotes cleanliness and prevents skin dryness or excessive moisture both of which predisposes to skin breakdown
Change socks daily; use loosely fitting warm cotton socks at night	Promotes warmth to feet and avoids fabrics that keep moisture in, such as synthetics
Trim toenails with clipper straight across and smooth with emery board; soak in warm water if nails are thick and hard	Prevents nail segment from penetrating groove as it grows and scratches from rough nails
Apply moleskin to corns and calluses	Decreases pressure and friction and protects lesions from injury

Information, Instruction, Demonstration

Interventions	Rationales
Advise to inspect skin daily or have someone else do it	Identifies irritations, inflammation or breaks in skin of feet
Instruct in daily foot care, proper socks, type of shoe to wear (oxford type or slip on with round toes and broad heels, long enough to extend 1½ inches beyond large toe)	Prevents infection, trauma and promotes mobility
Instruct in foot exercises: flex and extend toes and ankles, rotate feet clockwise and counter-clockwise	Promotes foot agility
Avoid use of commercial products for corns, calluses	Contains harsh chemicals which damage skin

Interventions	Rationales
Avoid use of heating pads, hot water bottles or packs on feet	May cause burns
Avoid trimming corns, calluses with sharp instruments	May nick skin and cause infection
Suggest use of podiatrist for foot care and nail trimming if unable to perform procedure	Improper care and trimming leads to foot problems especially if circulatory disorder present
Instruct in trimming nails using nailclip from side to middle of nail cutting straight across at proper length	Proper nail trimming will prevent ingrown nail and infection
Administration of antifungal drops or cream to nails	Destroys microorganisms causing infection

Discharge or Maintenance Evaluation

- Absence of inflammation, infection of nails or skin of feet
- Absence of breaks or cuts in skin
- Compliance with daily foot care, medication application
- Proper trimming and padding of nails and toes
- Visits to podiatrist for ongoing foot care
- Absence of complications resulting from corns, calluses, bunions or new buildup of kerotonic tissue

Psychosocial Considerations

Psychosocial Considerations

The consideration of mental and social health and function are facets of all problems in a holistic approach to the care of the elderly. They are interrelated with the physiological changes and problems of the group and require a special empathy and sensitivity to needs and feelings of each aging client. Some important mental and social health problems are anxiety, depression, dementia, loneliness, disengagement or withdrawn from family and social interaction, grief and retirement.

GENERAL PSYCHOSOCIAL CHANGES ASSOCIATED WITH THE AGING PROCESS

- Reduced functional reserve and adaptive capacity causing increased vulnerability to illness, multiple stressors associated with environmental and psychosocial changes
- Reduced integrative and regulatory mechanisms causing increased and inconsistent physiologic, mental and behavioral responses resulting in reduced ability to restore or maintain homeostasis
- Multisystem stressors causing reduced capacity to adapt
- Developmental task achievement causing positive adjustment and view of aging; coping with loss(es); development of new roles, skills, relationships; giving up of former power behaviors; adaptation to diminished health, social and economic resources

Combative, Disruptive Behavior

Disruptive/Combative Behavior

| ↓ | ↓ | ↓ | ↓ |

Dementia/confusion   Drug toxicity,   Neurosensory deficit   Dependency
Depression   withdrawal   Musculoskeletal   Loss of control
Isolation   impairment
Loneliness

| ↓ | ↓ | ↓ | ↓ |

Agitation
Aggressive/combative behavior
Verbal abuse (profanity, obscenities)
Physical abuse (biting, kicking, hitting)
Violence to self or others

Combative Disruptive Behavior

Any behavior that creates a disruptive environment by the elderly is considered disruptive or combative whether verbal or physical. It is usually directed at a family member or caregiver and may be triggered by physiological or psychological conditions.

MEDICAL CARE

Psychotherapeutics: haloperidol (Haldol), thiothixene (Navane) PO to act on all levels of CNS to depress all body functions to decrease displays of emotions and suppress spontaneous movement and complex behavior in agitated states

Electrolyte panel: Reveals abnormal levels of electrolytes or imbalances leading to agitation

Drug levels: Reveals toxic levels responsible for behavior changes

NURSING CARE PLANS

Essential nursing diagnoses and plans associated with this condition:

Sleep pattern disturbance (77)

Related to: Internal factors of illness, psychological stress, external factors of environmental changes
Defining characteristics: Interrupted sleep, increasing irritability, restlessness, listlessness, expressionless face

Risk for impaired skin integrity (246)

Related to: Internal factor of psychogenic self-inflicted injury
Defining characteristics: Scratches, hematomas, dry, itchy skin, falls, trauma, breaks in skin

Altered thought processes (70)

Related to: Psychological conflicts
Defining characteristics: Agitation, aggressiveness, confusion, inappropriate affect, verbal or physical abuse

SPECIFIC DIAGNOSES AND CARE PLANS

Risk for self or other directed violence

Related to: Toxic reaction to medications, dementia, loss of independence (disruptive/combative behavior)
Defining characteristics: Agitation, aggressive activity, violence to self or others, loss of control, depression, high level anxiety, physical abuse (biting, kicking, hitting), bruises, breaks in skin

Outcome Criteria

Control of disruptive/combative behavior.

Interventions	Rationales
Assess behavior pattern, ability to control behavior and express needs and feelings, demanding or withdrawn, refusing food, medication or assistance, agitation and combative actions	Identifies actual or potential violent behavior

Interventions	Rationales
Assess for expression of hopelessness and loss of desire to live	Indicates possible death wish and suicide attempt
Remove all sharp, unsafe articles from environment	May be used to inflict harm on self or others
Avoid rushing, abrupt changes in care or environment	Prevents frustration that results in agitation
Provide nonthreatening and nonjudgmental environment; interact with client as often as possible	Promotes trusting relationship and decreases abusive/disruptive behavior against caregiver
Maintain self-care practices with self-pacing by client; allow for freedom to control own care as appropriate	Maintains personal space and control over life
Avoid threats, arguing or questions when giving care or dealing with disruptive behavior	May cause threat and loss of control of behavior
Provide exercises and group activities; set aside times for acting-out behavior	Promotes socialization and diversion; allows for expression of feelings and frustrations
Avoid restraining or overmedicating unless harmful behavior uncontrollable	Further exacerbates agitation and disruptive behavior

Information, Instruction, Demonstration

Interventions	Rationales
Suggest music, pet therapy	Provides calming environment
Instruct in making simple decisions in daily routines and to allow for flexibility if needed	Promotes control over environment

Interventions	Rationales
Involve client in all planning of care	Promotes understanding of expected behaviors

Discharge or Maintenance Evaluation

- Client verbalizes methods to change or control behavior
- Disruptive episodes reduced or eliminated
- Environment safe for client and caregiver
- Absence of violence against self and others
- Participates in therapy to reduce agitation and aggressive behavior

Altered family processes

Related to: Situational crisis (disruptive behavior)
Defining characteristics: Family system unable to meet physical, emotional needs of client, inability to cope with disruptive behavior

Outcome Criteria

Improved understanding and coping ability of family.

Interventions	Rationales
Assess family knowledge of reasons for client behavior, possible violence, how to handle disruptive behavior	Knowledge will enhance family's understanding of the basis for the behavior and how to develop coping skills and strategies
Assist family to identify client's reactions and behaviors	Gives indication of onset of behavior in order to adjust environment reduce episodes
Assist family in defining problem and use of techniques to cope	Provides support for problem-solving and management of chronic stress and anxiety

Interventions	Rationales
Provide for opportunity of family to express concerns and lack of control of situation	Reduces anxiety and stress
Assist family to identify difference between intentional behaviors and those that are uncontrollable	Allows for appropriate responses to disruptive behavior

Information, Instruction, Demonstration

Interventions	Rationales
Instruct in importance and provision of safe environment for client and family	Prevents injury
Suggest day care, support groups for family	Provides respite from care of client and support and empathy
Inform of importance of continued visits and relationship with client	Prevents guilt feelings and disassociation of family
Instruct of need to maintain own health, social contacts	Physical and emotional health of family may be affected if own needs neglected

Discharge or Maintenance Evaluation

- Optimal health of family members
- Family participating in activities and maintaining social contacts
- Verbalization of understanding client's behavior, coping and problem-solving techniques utilized
- Uses support resources provided by community/private professionals
- Refrains from physical or verbal abuse directed at client

Depression

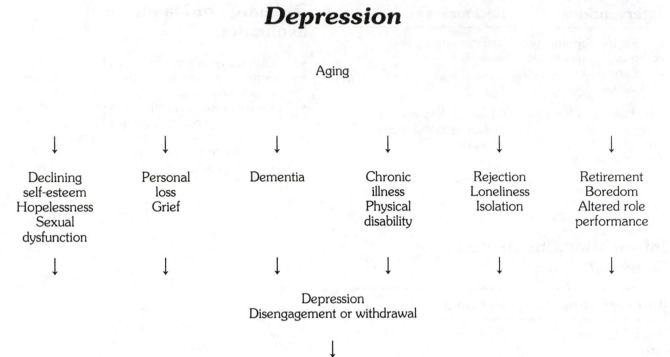

Aging

↓	↓	↓	↓	↓	↓
Declining self-esteem Hopelessness Sexual dysfunction	Personal loss Grief	Dementia	Chronic illness Physical disability	Rejection Loneliness Isolation	Retirement Boredom Altered role performance
↓	↓	↓	↓	↓	↓

Depression
Disengagement or withdrawal

↓

Suicide risk

Depression

Depression in the elderly is identified as a lowered mood disorder and a lack of psychic energy that is experienced by a client and either reported or observed. Types of depression affecting the elderly are masked depression (states that are missed as depression because the behavior does not typically resemble that of a younger depressed person or is written off in the elderly as uncooperative or irritability), reactive depression (states that are response to stimuli) and depressive states associated with dementia (chronic brain syndrome). Depression is the most prevelant psychological problem in the elderly and its frequency and acuteness increase with age. This is caused by the increase in the risk factors associated with depression in the elderly, i.e., loss and grief, hopelessness, helplessness, decreased self-esteem, isolation, apathy, diseases associated with dementia, sexual dysfunction, medication regimen, chronic illness.

MEDICAL CARE

Antidepressants (monamine oxidase inhibitors): phenelzine (Nardil), isocarboxazid (Marplan) PO to prevent breakdown of monoamines

Antidepressants (serotonin selective reuptake inhibitors): fluoxetine (Prozac), sertraline (Zoloft) PO to block reuptake of serotonin in CNS

Antidepressants (tricylics): trazodone (Desyrel), nortriptyline (Pamelor) PO to potentiate the effect of norepinephrine an serotonin in the treatment of depression in conjunction with psychotherapy

CT scan: Reveals underlying cause associated with dementia

Electrolyte panel: Reveals metabolic changes associated with depression

Electroencephalogum: reveals brain waves associated with depressive states

Dexamethasone suppression (DST): Reveals positive result if depression present

Medication levels: Reveals toxicity and possible cause of depression

NURSING CARE PLANS

Essential nursing diagnoses and plans associated with this condition:

Altered nutrition: less than body requirements (118)

Related to: Inability to ingest food because of psychological factor
Defining characteristics: Anorexia, lack of interest in food, apathy, weight loss, withdrawn, isolation

Sexual dysfunction (181)

Related to: Biopsychosocial alteration of sexuality from lack of significant other, altered body structure or function
Defining characteristics: Verbalization of problem, depression, chronic illness, grief, change in interest in self and others, inability to achieve desired satisfaction

Constipation (121)

Related to: Less than adequate intake of bulk and fluids, less that adequate physical activity, emotional status from depressive state
Defining characteristics: Hard-formed stool, less frequent stool passage, palpable mass, decreased appetite

Impaired verbal communication (75)

Related to: Psychological barriers from depression
Defining characteristics: Slowed speech, inability to find words

Sleep pattern disturbance (77)

Related to: Psychological stress from depression
Defining characteristics: Interrupted sleep, insomnia, early morning awakening, difficulty falling asleep, increasing irritability

Altered thought processes (70)

Related to: Psychological conflicts from depression
Defining characteristics: Retardation of thought, agitation, mood reactive or not reactive to environment, sadness, guilt, self-blame or blame on others, delusions, inappropriate affect, non-reality based thinking, despair

SPECIFIC DIAGNOSES AND CARE PLANS

Risk for self-directed violence

Related to: Suicidal behavior (depression over chronic, painful illness or loss
Defining characteristics: Inability to resolve depression, loneliness, social isolation, verbalized feelings of hopelessness, inability to cope, formulated plans for suicide, past attempts at suicide, cues or warning behavior of intentions

Outcome Criteria

Suicide attempt prevented.

Interventions	Rationales
Assess length and extent/depth of depression, reasons for depression, screen for symptoms using the Beck Depression Inventory or Geriatric Depression Scale	Depression is predisposing to and increases risk for suicide in the elderly
Assess whether client has considered suicide, thought about it, has a plan for suicide	Places client at higher risk for suicide potential; the more thought out the intent and plan, the higher the risk
Assess for refusal to eat, hoarding of medication, refusing medications or other treatment	May indicate suicide potential
Administer antidepressants	Acts as mood elevator to treat depression
Discuss need to speak with a therapist or other resource person before committing suicide	Offers support to reverse decision and discuss other alternatives
Observe carefully for behavior indicative of suicide and remove dangerous items that could be used to injure the client (guns, knives, razor blades, ropes, medications, matches)	Provides safe environment and prevents self-directed injury
Encourage expression of feelings of anger, anxiety, guilt, fear, shame, loneliness, hopelessness, rejection, isolation	Promotes venting of feelings and may prevent suicide attempt
Assist to explore reasons for wanting to end life and life-events that lead the client to want to commit suicide	Assists to identify cause and issues related to problems that result in suicide attempt in order to resolve them

Interventions	Rationales
Encourage music therapy, relaxation techniques, reminiscence	Promotes diversional relaxation and review thoughts about accomplishments, unresolved conflicts, life events all of which assists to integrate life losses and failures with accomplishments and positive past experiences

Information, Instruction, Demonstration

Interventions	Rationales
Suggest referral to therapy with gero-psychiatrist or other counseling as appropriate	Assists to overcome depression and develop skills in coping and problem-solving
Instruct to call therapist or other help such as hotlines before attempting suicide	Provides expression of feelings and opportunity to reconsider options
Instruct family or caregiver of behaviors indicating risk for suicide	Provides warning signals before suicide attempt is made
Inform that at least 4 weeks needed for medication results	Time is needed for optimal effect

Discharge or Maintenance Evaluation

- Suicide attempt prevented
- Verbalizes awareness of reasons for depression and risk for suicide and what to do before an attempt is made
- Uses support systems offered by group therapy, psychotherapy with therapist
- Participates in music and/or reminiscent therapy

- Absence of suicidal behavior and consideration of suicide as way to solve problems

Social isolation

Related to: Alterations in mental status (depression)
Defining characteristics: Sad, dull affect, uncommunicative, withdrawn, expresses feeling of aloneness, rejection, grief, loss(es), absence of supportive significant other(s), inability to meet expectations of others, indifference by others, or lack of support system

Outcome Criteria

Return to or maintenance of social relationships.

Interventions	Rationales
Assess feelings about behavioral problems, negative feelings about self, ability to communicate, anxiety, depression, feeling of powerlessness	Determines extent of loneliness, isolation and reasons for depression
Assist to identify barriers to developing relationships and participating in activities	Understanding reasons for isolation provides motivation for resolving it
Provide encouragement and positive reinforcement for any behavior indicating renewed interest in social participation	Promotes reduction of social isolation and supports social interaction to reduce loneliness and depression
Provide diversional activities as appropriate to functional (physical and psychological) abilities	Provides stimuli and promotes psychosocial functioning
Assist to identify possible support systems (clergy, therapist, telephone); strategies to overcome obstacles	Promotes return to and new relationships and development of new interests

Information, Instruction, Demonstration

Interventions	Rationales
Offer list of available resources for assistance and social opportunities, therapy as appropriate (cognitive, behavior, music or reminisient therapy)	Provides social outlet, counseling and other assists if needed
Suggest volunteer programs for participation, community centers for older adults	Provides social interaction and satisfaction

Discharge or Maintenance Evaluation

- Verbalizes establishment of meaningful relationships, friendships
- Verbalizes a decrease in loneliness, distrust
- Some degree of lifting of depression
- Develops interest and participation in community or volunteer activities
- Participates in group support services or individual counseling to reduce depression

Grief

Normal bereavement following the death of a loved one occurs over time with movement through the grieving process in an individual manner. The process of handling grief may be called "grief work." It may be acute (following a sudden unanticipated loss) or chronic (prolonged and intense over a limited or expanded time as in the deterioration of a loved one). Anticipatory grief identifies preparatory and premourning activities and a morbid grief reaction is the distortion of of grieving by prolonged and excessive preoccupation with grief work. As one ages, loss becomes an inevitable occurrence as it includes loss of independence and competence through increasing frailty and disabilities through illnesses such as stroke, COPD and loss of spouse, friends, relatives and material possessions such as a home. The grieving process may be associated with any loss of cumulative losses experienced by the older adult and expressions of sadness and grief which are unique to an individual should be allowed in a supportive, nonjudgemental environment.

NURSING CARE PLANS

Essential nursing diagnoses and plans associated with this condition:

Sleep pattern disturbance (77)

Related to: Psychological stress from loss
Defining characteristics: Verbal complaints of not feeling well rested, interrupted sleep, insomnia, irritability, lethargy, lake of energy

SPECIFIC DIAGNOSES AND CARE PLANS

Spiritual distress (distress of the human spirit)

Related to: Challenged belief and value system (result of therapy or intense suffering, loss of loved one)
Defining characteristics: Questions meaning of suffering, verbalizes inner conflicts about beliefs, questions moral and ethical implications of therapeutic regimen, regards illness as punishment, description of somatic complaints, alterations in behavior or mood (anger, crying, anxiety, hostility, apathy, withdrawal, preoccupation)

Outcome Criteria

Resolution of spiritual well-being.

Interventions	Rationales
Assess expression of religious views, affiliation, ways of dealing with spiritual needs and rituals of importance, personal difficulties with religious beliefs	Provides information to assist in reconciling beliefs and demise; majority of elderly have religious affiliation which offers source of support, meaning to life and identity
Assess for dissatisfaction with own care during illness or care of deceased loved one	Provides information about feelings associated with care and/or limitations in practices with respect to care
Assess for ability to interact and ask questions	Promotes assistance in resolution of moral/ethical conflicts
Communicate respect for client's religious beliefs	Promotes understanding and trusting relationship

Grief

Aging

↓   ↓   ↓

Loss of loved one   Life threatening   Chronic disease
Loss of possession   illness of loved one   Disability
↓   ↓   ↓

Grief   ←

Reduced self-esteem, anticipatory grief

↓

Sadness, regret
Guilt, ambivalence
Loneliness
Emotional, physical pain
↓

Stages of brieving (grief work)
(shock, disbelief, denial, anger,
guilt and depression, resolution
and acceptance)
↓

Renewed acquaintances
and activities
Adjustment to a new lifestyle

Interventions	Rationales
Encourage and accept verbal responses of anger, hostility and other behavior alterations	Promotes venting of feelings in accepting, nonjudgemental environment without more guilt and shame
Provide prayer times, times for religious rituals	Promotes religious faith and support

Information, Instruction, Demonstration

Interventions	Rationales
Inform of availability of services and visits from clergy or spiritual counseling	Promotes religious practices and support
Instruct in values clarification, imagery, music therapy	Promotes comfort with beliefs, diversion and relaxation

Discharge or Maintenance Evaluation

- Client verbalizes positive statements about self and life
- Develops own religious support system
- Able to articulate how religious beliefs fit into lifestyle and/or assists in coping with loss or illness
- Uses spiritual professional assistance, techniques to deal with illness and/or loss

Ineffective individual coping

Related to: Situational crises (loss), chronic illness
Defining characteristics: Death of spouse, family member, loss of independence and control, disability, chronic illness, impaired social interaction, participation, verbalization of inability to cope or ask for help to meet basic needs, inappropriate use of defense

mechanisms, chronic fatigue, insomnia, anorexia, headache, chronic worry, anxiety, chronic depression

Outcome Criteria

Improved psychological and social coping skills.

Interventions	Rationales
Assess expressions of anxiety, depression, loneliness, hopelessness, social isolation over loss	Successful coping with loss and ability to develop compensatory behaviors to adjust to changes affecting development task accomplishment in the elderly and their ability to cope
Assess use of coping skills, ability to cope with losses, fear of own death, chronic worry and anxiety	The elderly have outstanding coping ability and adaptability although loss may tax their adaptive mechanisms and ability to respond and maintain a balance to homeostasis
Assist to identify positive defense mechanisms and promote their use	Use of defense mechanisms that have worked in the past increase ability to cope and move through grieving process
Provide environment that allows for free expression of concerns and fears, mourning responses	Encourages trust and relieves anxiety and worry, guilt and sadness

Information, Instruction, Demonstration

Interventions	Rationales
Social and coping skills with problem-solving approaches	Prevents disengagement and promotes coping ability with lifestyle changes

Interventions	Rationales
New ways or methods to adapt roles to new situation or needs	Provides for alternatives if usual mechanisms are not satisfactory
Suggest support group or counseling if appropriate	Provides information and support for changes and adaptation skills

Discharge or Maintenance Evaluation

- Verbalizes that anxiety and fear reduced
- Uses appropriate old or new coping and problem-solving skills in adapting to illness, loss
- Asks for and utilizes assistance when needed
- Increased participation in new roles, skills, social activities

Dysfunctional grieving

Related to: Loss of significant other, personal possessions; chronic fatal illness
Defining characteristics: Verbal expression of distress at loss, expression of guilt, self-blame, unresolved issues, anger, sadness, crying, denial of loss, difficulty in expressing loss, altered eating, sleeping, dreaming, activity, libido patterns, reliving of past experiences, labile affect, alterations in concentration and/or pursuit of tasks, interference with life-functioning

Outcome Criteria

Progressive resolution of grieving process.

Interventions	Rationales
Assess for stage in grieving process, personal strengths and inner resources that assist in coping with actual loss	Stages are normal responses leading to acceptance and resolution of loss

Interventions	Rationales
Assist to differentiate between helpful or maladaptive use of denial and reinforcement of this behavior; prolonged time spent in other stages of grieving	Although sometimes stages display some overlapping in behaviors, prolonged maladaptive use of behaviors or mechanisms prevent movement through the grieving process and may result in delayed or morbid grief reaction
Provide environment and conducive to expressions of hostility, guilt, sorrow, sense of loss, feelings of ambivalence	Provides openness supportive environment for grief management
Assist client to understand reasons for feelings, responses from others	Promotes understanding of behavior during grief work
Provide quiet and privacy when needed or requested; music therapy	Allows for thoughtful contemplation and reminiscence; music therapy provides communication, self-expression, improved motivation and pleasure for those suffering loss
Recognize and respect religious, economic, cultural aspects of client's grief	Promotes self-worth and positive, trusting relationship

Information, Instruction, Demonstration

Interventions	Rationales
Stages of grieving process, need to progress through each stage (grief work)	Normal grieving is a universal need and understanding of the stages; promotes resolution and self-confidence in grieving

Interventions	Rationales
Importance of communication with family/support systems	Promotes support at most critical times
Communicate information honestly when clarifying and presenting factual information in a realistic non-threatening fashion	Promotes trusting relationship and presents significant facts in a constructive manner
Inform of referrals for counseling or assistance in planning for future	Provides support and assistance if grief work not progressing or unresolved, potential for suicide, functional impairment, or feelings of worthlessness

Discharge or Maintenance Evaluation

- Able to discuss feelings regarding loss
- Maintains significant relationships and support systems during grieving process
- Identifies positive and negative behaviors and responses and promotes positive ones
- Seeks counseling assistance if appropriate

Recreation/Activiies

Aging

| ↓ | ↓ | ↓ | ↓ |

Retirement
Role change

Cognitive/
motor deficits

Chronic
illness

Socialization

| ↓ | ↓ | ↓ | ↓ |

Leasure time
Hobbies
Sports
Interests

Rehabilitation therapies

Unpaired social
interactions
Disengagement
or isolation

↓

Occupational
Physical
Speech
Pulmonary
Cardiac

| ↓ | ↓ | ↓ |

Group or individual activities
Structured activities to address special needs

Recreation/ Activities

Varied activities or services available to the older adult population provide and promote the health, contentment, and daily feeling of well-being. They stimulate the physical, mental, and social functions of the individual by providing therapeutic recreation, social activities, and facilitating interactions. Examples of group or individual activities include physical, sensory stimulating, spiritual, cognitive, emotionally supportive, educational, creative, social, self-expression and personal responsibility. Where deficits are present, they can be encouraged and/or supplemented by special therapy (physical, occupational, speech, recreational). Individual preferences and choices based on interests and needs must be considered to comply with satisfactory participation in structured or unstructured activities.

NURSING CARE PLANS

Essential nursing diagnoses and plans associated with this condition:

Impaired physical mobility (196)

Related to: Intolerance to activity; decreased strength and endurance
Defining characteristics: Decreased muscle strength, control, and/or mass, limited range of motion

Risk for trauma (198)

Related to: Internal factors of weakness, lack of safety precautions, cognitive or emotional difficulties
Defining characteristics: Poor sensory perception (vision, auditory, tactile), balancing difficulty, motor incoordination, unsafe recreational/activity environment, anxiety, apathy

Sensory/perceptual alterations (visual, auditory, tactile) (72)

Related to: Altered sensory reception, transmission, and/or integration, aging process
Defining characteristics: Disorientation, depression, mood swings, poor concentration, restlessness, irritability, lack of concentration

SPECIFIC DIAGNOSES AND CARE PLANS

Diversional activity deficit

Related to: Environmental lack of diversional activity
Defining characteristics: Boredom, desire for something interesting to do, unable to select preferred activities, lack of assistance needed to engage in activities, poor scheduling of activities, insufficient equipment/supplies and space to perform activities, sensory and motor deficits, refusal to participate in activities

Outcome Criteria

Adapts and participates in diversional activities available and related to interests and health status

Interventions	Rationales
Assess for therapeutic recreation or activities such as physical, sensory stimulating, spiritual, cognitive, educational, creative, social activities and those that offer emotional support and allow for self-expression, personal responsibility and choice	Special needs can be addressed by services designed to meet interests and well-being of individuals

Interventions	Rationales
Provide written choices that include a schedule of hobbies, dance, drama, music, exercise, current events, Bible study, book reviews, reminiscence, care of pets, arts and crafts, cooking	Offers structured or unstructured group or individual activities planned by a recreation therapist
Provide assistive devices if deficits present	Assists to manage and support activity
Include qualified personnel based on individual needs such as therapists for speech, skills, sensory stimulation	Provides direction and supervision of activities prescribed for special rehabilitation fine and gross motor needs
Introduce to new activities and resources, new acquaintances or groups	Promotes social interactions and motivates group process
Promote a friendly accepting attitude among participants	Promotes group discussions and comments and ideas from each member

Information, Instruction, Demonstration

Interventions	Rationales
Formulate activity schedule times and type and setting and allow to review and select those for participation	Promotes choice of activities based on interests
Inform of importance of remaining active and involved in various leisure or recreational activities	Promotes personal satisfaction as physical and, sometimes, mental deterioration decline
Involve in making selections that fit interests and daily routines	Promotes control over environment

Interventions	Rationales
Inform of safety hazards involved in activities and utilizes aids or accepts assistance when necessary	Maintains safe environment, prevents injury

Discharge or Maintenance Evaluation

- Uses resources (special equipment) available to participate in therapeutic activities
- Interacts positively with others, attends group activities
- Avoids social isolation and develops and maintains relationships
- Chooses time and number of activities and changes activity participation if desired or needed
- Reflects interest and enjoyment for activities

Retirement

Retirement is the termination of an occupational career and a process that includes adjustment to a social role with rights, duties and relationships with others in the environment. General expectations of the retired elderly by society are to manage their own life and live within their income, to remain the same type of person as they were before retirement (ways of thinking, general mannerisms and job skills) and to stay out of the job market and select volunteer and leisure roles instead. Consequences of retirement may be changes in and eligibility for other roles, identity crisis, change and increase in social participation and leisure pursuits, poverty, housing in retirement villages or other changes in residence. In general, retirement does not have negative consequences for health, social life or self-esteem unless the individual is already in poor health, experiences multiple role losses or was overinvolved in their job and never developed a range of leisure activities and skills.

MEDICAL CARE

Anxiolytics: alprazolam (Xanax), brazepam (Ativan) PO for short term treatment of anxiety by depressing effect on subcortical levels of CNS and action on limbic system

NURSING CARE PLANS

Essential nursing diagnoses and plans associated with this condition:

Impaired physical mobility (196)

Related to: Intolerance to activity, severe anxiety, musculoskeletal or neuromuscular impairment
Defining characteristics: Inability to participate in leisure activities, anxiety caused by retirement, reduced health, energy and neurosensory function

SPECIFIC DIAGNOSES AND CARE PLANS

Anxiety

Related to: Change in role functioning and socio-economic status; maturational crisis (retirement)
Defining characteristics: Feelings of inadequacy, uncertainty, apprehension, tension about retirement and changes in lifestyle, insomnia, depression

Outcome Criteria

Reduced anxiety within manageable levels.

Interventions	Rationales
Assess feelings associated with retirement, ability to adapt to new lifestyle and role changes, pre-retirement plans	Retirement can result in anxiety if sudden or void of plans for this developmental stage in life
Assess for signs and symptoms of anxiety and determine if mild, moderate or severe	Reveals severity of impact of retirement on individual
Assess for phase of retirement and motivation to achieve meaningful retirement	May hide behind sick role as way to deal with fear of retirement as an unknown
Assess effect of retirement on health, self-esteem, social participation, living accommodations and economic resources	Source of anxiety in retired persons
Provide time for listening in a nonjudgemental environment	Promotes venting of feeling to reduce anxiety

Information, Instruction, Demonstration

Interventions	Rationales
Refer to support groups or counseling as appropriate	Provides support for task achievement of retirement
Relaxation exercises and techniques, guided imagery, music	Relieves anxiety

Discharge or Maintenance Evaluation

- Verbalizes a reduction in anxiety
- Uses techniques to relieve anxiety
- Progressive movement in acceptance of and adaptation to retirement states

Diversional activity deficit

Related to: Environmental lack of diversional activity (retirement)
Defining characteristics: Boredom, excessive amount of leisure time, lack of financial resources, lack of interest in recreational activities, impaired health, chronic illness, lack of development of leisure interests and activities

Outcome Criteria

Adjustment to retirement and increased leisure within limitations.

Interventions	Rationales
Assess feelings about retirement, attitudes toward leisure and interests in recreational participation	An increase in leisure time in retirement may cause problems in those who have not been involved in activities and developed leisure skills

Interventions	Rationales
Suggest recreational facilities, programs, community centers that provide leisure activities, fitness programs	Day centers, community elderly programs are available and promote activities and socialization regardless of financial ability
Suggest volunteer roles that provide accomplishment and enhance self-worth	Some volunteer roles are menial and depreciating and provide little satisfaction for a retiree
Promote leisure activities such as reading, TV, radio, listening to tapes, CDs, playing games (cards, Bingo, Scrabble)	Provides leisure activities for those who are homebound or have limited physical and economic resources
Encourage to participate in former away from home activities (golf, travel, tennis, bridge contests, concerts, fairs, exhibits)	Maintains social relationships and continues with established leisure interests

Information, Instruction, Demonstration

Interventions	Rationales
Inform of new daily activities and assist with planning	Promotes leisure time for those who have not developed leisure skills
Provide list of agencies, community resources that provide leisure activities	Allows for independent selection of activities

Discharge or Maintenance Evaluation

- Learns and uses new leisure skills
- Participates in leisure activities of choice
- Verbalizes that adjusting to retirement and additional time for leisure
- Maintains social interaction and participation within limitations

General Considerations

Malignancies and Chemotherapy/ Radiotherapy

Malignancy, also known as carcinoma or cancer, is a tumor that invades surrounding tissue with the capability of spreading to tissues at distant site(s) in the body (metastasis). This unregulated cell destruction is the result of uncontrolled and abnormal cell growth. Any system can be affected by solid tumor organ sites or blood-forming organ sites. Physical changes resulting from the disease process and treatments as well as psychosocial responses to the disease have an impact on the client's life. These are the basis for nursing care planning for all malignancies regardless of organs or systems. Cancer is a leading cause of death in the elderly and the most common malignancies in the older adult are lung, colorectal, breast, prostate, leukemia, and lymphoma.

MEDICAL CARE

Analgesics: oxycodone (Percodan), codeine (Methylmorphine) PO and morphine (MS), meperidine (Demeral) IM single dose or fentanyl (Duragesic) continuous by client-controlled device (PCA) depending on pain assessment for pain relief by decreasing neurotransmitter release resulting in analgesia

Chemotherapy: Protocol of antineoplastic drug combinations to manage solid tumor growth, lymphomas, and leukemias, and their metastasis to other organ systems; can be given with other treatments such as radiotherapy and surgery. Selections based on type and extent of the disease and include alkylating

agents, antimetabolites, antitumor antibotics and anthracyclines, enzymes, hormones, vinca alkaloids, antiproliferative, immunotherapy, and others

Antianxiety agent: alprazolam (Xanax) PO to relieve anxiety by depressive action on many levels of CNS

Antiemetic: prochlorperazine (Compazine), benzquinamide (Emete-con) PO prior to and following therapy to relieve nausea and vomiting

Antidiarrheal: diphenoxylate/atropine (Lomotil), kaolin/pectin (Kaotin) to relieve diarrhea resulting from therapy by decreasing bowel motility and feces water content

Astringent: chlorhexidine gluconate or Domboro solution as cleansing agent to treat desquamation caused by external radiation therapy

Prostate specific antigen (PSA): Diagnostic for prostate cancer

Carcinoembryonic antigen enzyme (CEA): Reveals high titers in extensive invasion of tumor with return to normal following surgery

Complete blood count (CBC): Reveals abnormal level of counts affected by disease or therapy (RBC, WBC, platelets)

Sputum or bronchial washings: Cytology studies reveal malignant cells

Feces analysis: Reveals occult blood indicating possible colorectal cancer

Bone marrow aspiration: Reveals abnormalities indicating leukemia

Chest and bone x-rays: Reveals lung involvement and aids in staging process; bone metastasis if present with osteoblastic changes

Mammography: Reveals lesion prior to surgery or in remaining breast

Bronchoscopy: Views area diagnosis, for tumor excision or biopsy

Colonoscopy/Proctosigmoidoscopy: Reveals polyp/tumor location and removal or biopsy

Barium enema: Reveals tumor site

Tissue biopsies: Excision or needle biopsy specimen from breast, lung, prostate, lymph node, colon revealing infiltration, cancer cells or to stage a tumor

Radionuclide scans: Computerized scanning following an IV injection of a radionuclide specific to organ uptake for presence of tumor

External radiation: May be done as the primary treatment to destroy tumor, adjunct therapy to surgery or chemotherapy to prevent recurrence or shrink tumor to size that is operable, or palliation of symptom of pain depending on tumor staging

Surgery: Prostatectomy with or without radical resection, bilateral orchiectomy in advanced stage; pneumonectomy, lobectomy to remove tumor; removal of tumor with right or left colectomy with anastomosis, abdominoperineal resection with permanent colostomy; lumpectomy, simple, modified radical, radical mastectomy depending on need for biopsy, tumor removal, or staging of disease

NURSING CARE PLANS

Essential nursing diagnoses and plans associated with these conditions:

Ineffective breathing pattern (45)

Related to: Pain of tumor invasion, decreased energy and fatigue from treatment regimen
Defining characteristics: Respiratory depth changes, inability to cough up secretions

Related to: Inflammatory process of disease
Defining characteristics: Tachypnea, dyspnea, cough

Related to: Decreased lung expansion
Defining characteristics: Dyspnea, effect of analgesia, respiratory depth changes

Related to: Tracheobronchial obstruction by tumor
Defining characteristics: Tachypnea, dyspnea, use of accessory muscles, respiratory depth changes, rhonchi, crackles, excessive mucus production, stasis of secretions, bronchial obstruction by tumor mass

Risk for fluid volume deficit (151)

Related to: Excessive losses through normal route associated with chemotherapy/radiotherapy
Defining characteristics: Nausea, vomiting, thirst, dry skin and mucous membranes, concentrated urine, diarrhea

Fluid volume excess (8)

Related to: Compromised regulatory mechanism resulting from radical surgery and removal of or irradiation of lymph nodes
Defining characteristics: Lymphedema in arm on affected side, heaviness, pain, impaired motor function, numbness and paresthesias of fingers

Diarrhea (121)

Related to: Medications and/or radiation to treat tumor causing inflammation of the bowel mucosa
Defining characteristics: Frequent, loose feces, cramping, abdominal pain, increased bowel sounds

Altered oral mucous membrane

Related to: Infection/inflammation resulting from chemotherapy/radiotherapy
Defining characteristics: Oral pain or discomfort, mucositis, stomatitis

Sexual dysfunction (181)

Related to: Biophysical alteration caused by altered body structure of function resulting from radical surgery or radiotherapy

Defining characteristics: Erectile dysfunction, impotence, verbalization of the inability to achieve sexual satisfaction, anxiety, limitations imposed by hormone therapy or surgery (colostomy, prostatectomy, orchiectomy)

Sleep pattern disturbance (77)

Related to: Internal factor of serious illness
Defining characteristics: Pain, dyspnea, lethargy, restlessness, interrupted sleep

SPECIFIC DIAGNOSES AND CARE PLANS

Anxiety

Related to: Threat of death (presence of cancer, uncertain prognosis)
Defining characteristics: Communication of fear and apprehension uncertainty of treatment regimen and outcome

Related to: Change in health status (effect of therapy and disease on lifestyle)
Defining characteristics: Communication of increased helplessness, dependence on others

Outcome Criteria

Reduced anxiety within manageable levels.

Interventions	Rationales
Assess facial expressions, restlessness, focus on self, avoidance of eye contact, tremors, quivering voice, perspiration	Objective signs of anxiety become more obvious as anxiety increases
Assess expressed feelings of tension, fear, uncertainty, response to diagnosis and treatments	Subjective signs of anxiety that reveal severity of impact of illness on patient

Interventions	Rationales
Provide quiet, nonjudgmental environment; allow for expression of fears and concerns about diagnosis and treatment	Promotes trusting relationship and reduces anxiety
Provide time to listen and answer questions simply and honestly or acquire information if needed	Promotes communication and relieves anxiety caused by unknowns

Information, Instruction, Demonstration

Interventions	Rationales
Relaxation exercises, guided imagery, music	Provides distractions and reduces anxiety
Suggest contact with clergy, counseling service or support group if need is felt	Provides support and spiritual guidance to reduce anxiety

Discharge or Maintenance Evaluation

- Verbalizes decreased anxiety
- States how condition will affect lifestyle
- Verbalizes uncertainty and apprehension has decreased with information and/or relaxation techniques

Anticipatory grieving

Related to: Perceived potential loss of physio-psychosocial well-being (potential death from fatal illness)
Defining characteristics: Expression of distress at potential loss, guilt, anger, sorrow

Outcome Criteria

Progressive movement through stages of grieving.

Interventions	Rationales
Assess stage of grieving process experienced; feelings about diagnosis	Stages are normal responses leading to acceptance of loss and include shock and disbelief, anger, depression
Assess presence of denial, guilt, anger, sadness	Normal responses to grief associated with fatal illness
Provide opportunity for expressing emotions related to anticipated loss	Allows for venting of feelings
Be honest in communications, acknowledge reality of fears expressed	Promotes trusting relationship
Identify support system of family, significant other, clergy	Positive support system and feelings for relationships enhance movement through grieving process
Encourage maintenance of rest, nutrition, activity needs	Promotes continous self-care
Provide quiet and privacy when requested	Allows for thoughtful relaxation
Recognize and respect religious, economic, educational, and cultural aspects of patient	Promotes sense of identity and positive self worth

Information, Instruction, Demonstration

Interventions	Rationales
Stages of grieving process, need to progress through each stage	Provides more understanding of behaviors in grieving
Importance of communication with family/support systems	Promotes needed support at most critical times

Discharge or Maintenance Evaluation

- Able to discuss feelings regarding anticipated loss
- Maintains significant relationships and support systems
- Maintains self-care and basic needs
- Identifies plans for changes in lifestyle and potential premature death

Pain

Related to: Biological injuring agents (tumor invasion, compression)
Defining characteristics: Communication of pain descriptors

Related to: Physical injuring agents (external radiation)
Defining characteristics: Communication of pain descriptors, guarding behavior, protective of radiated site

Outcome Criteria

Relief and control of pain.

Interventions	Rationales
Assess pain for severity, intermittent or persistent in area	Result of liberation of pain mediators by tumor, tumor compression and ischemia of structures
Assess pain in irradiated area depending on amount and frequency of doses	Result of inflammation of irradiated area, exposure of nerve endings in area
Administer analgesic SC, IM; usually on demand, self-operated syringe infusion pump device	Relieves pain that becomes increasingly severe
Maintain irradiated area clean and dry; avoid removing any markings when cleansing	Reduces pain in presence of moist desquamation

Interventions	Rationales
Cover irradiated area with dressing	Prevents exposure to air which increases pain in area
Assist to or change position using pillows, gentle, smooth movements	Promotes comfort and relieves pressure that causes pain
Massage back, extremities	Promotes comfort and relaxation
Remain when requested and use therapeutic touch if appropriate	Give comfort and reassurance, displays caring

Information, Instruction, Demonstration

Interventions	Rationales
Administration of analgesic therapy; use of infusion device	Assists to control pain and provide safe analgesic therapy
Expected effect of medications and need for reporting pain that is not controlled	Offers opportunity to change medication

Discharge or Maintenance Evaluation

- Statement that pain is absent with maintenance of continuous state of comfort
- Analgesic effective in controlling pain with minimal side effects
- Relaxed expression, able to rest without complaints of pain

Fatigue

Related to: Overwhelming psychological or emotional demands (cancer and treatment regimen)
Defining characteristics: Verbalization of fatigue/lack of energy, inability to maintain usual routines, decreased performance, emotionally labile or irritable

Related to: States of discomfort (pain, treatment regimen, dypnea)
Defining characteristics: Increase in physical complaints

Outcome Criteria

Increased activity tolerance and energy level within illness limitations.

Interventions	Rationales
Assess activity tolerance, sleep pattern, anxiety	Determines baseline for activity limitations to prevent fatigue
Assist to plan schedule of paced activities, rest, exercise within tolerance level	Maintains activity while preventing fatigue
Provide quiet, stress-free environment	Promotes rest and prevents anxiety resulting from increased stimuli
Assist with ADL as needed with consideration for personal requests and desires	Conserves energy; prevents fatigue caused by destruction of normal and abnormal cells by chemotherapy and radiation

Information, Instruction, Demonstration

Interventions	Rationales
Avoid activities beyond level of tolerance; ask for assistance when needed	Conserves energy
Place articles within reach, use energy saving devices when possible	Prevents unnecessary activity and fatigue

Interventions	Rationales
Importance of rest, nutrition and exercise	Maintains basic needs necessary to prevent fatigue
Fatigue increases as disease and treatment regimen progresses	Anemia results from chemotherapy and reduces activity tolerance

Discharge or Maintenance Evaluation

- Minimal fatigue level associated with activity limitations
- Statements of interest in activity and fatigue reduced
- Able to participate in activity with performance limited to activity tolerance

Altered nutrition: less than body requirements

Related to: Inability to ingest food because of biological factors (chemotherapy/radiation)
Defining characteristics: Loss of weight; 20% or more under ideal weight, reported inadequate food intake, sore, inflamed buccal cavity, anorexia, nausea, vomiting

Outcome Criteria

Adequate nutritional intake with weight at baseline level for height and frame.

Interventions	Rationales
Assess weight loss, weakness, tissue/muscle wasting, cachexia	Results from catabolic effect of tumor on body metabolism and trapping of nutrients by rapidly dividing tumor cells

Interventions	Rationales
Assess degree of anorexia, nausea, vomiting, presence of stomatitis, mucositis, dyspepsia, dysphagia	Associated with chemotherapy/radiation affecting oral and gastrointestinal mucosa
Assess amount, types of food eaten compared to calorie needs that will maintain weight	Assists to determine menus that will provide adequate nutritional intake
Administer antiemetic PO promethazine (Phenergan), dronabinol (Marinol); may be administrated 12 hours before therapy and q4-6 hours before and after therapy	Reduces nausea and vomiting by depressing chemoreceptor trigger zone (CTZ) in medulla
Administer IV chemotherapy before time of sleep and give slowly	Prevents opportunity for nausea if asleep and decreases stimulation of vomiting center
Offer 6 small meals/day of high protein, caloric food selections; supplement with Ensure or other high caloric beverage as desired	Reduces fatigue, high protein and caloric intake for cell building and maintaining weight with increased metabolism
Offer wine, brandy, soft foods such as custards, Jello; suggest eating slowly and chewing foods well; drink fluids during meals to moisten foods	Stimulates appetite and increases intake if stomatitis, dysphagia present
Maintain clean, odor free environment	Improves desire to eat
Change positions slowly and elevate head of bed after eating	Prevents stimulation of chemoreceptor trigger zone that causes vomiting
Provide oral care before and after eating; mouthwash q2-4h with saline, baking soda and water, hydrogen peroxide solution	Prevents nausea and vomiting; treats impaired oral mucosa caused by breakdown of oral epithelial cells

Interventions	Rationales
Apply topical anesthetics (viscous xylocaine), artificial saliva (Salivart)	Allays oral mucosa pain, prevents dryness and breakdown of oral mucosa by lubrication
Remove dentures except for eating	Prevents further irritation to sore oral mucosa

Information, Instruction, Demonstration

Interventions	Rationales
Avoid hot, spicy foods, foods that are acidic	Irritating to inflamed oral and gastrointestinal mucosa
Include bland foods and drinks, thickened foods, cool drinks such as popsicles, milkshakes, cream or pureed foods	Soothes mucosa and provides foods and drinks that are easily swallowed
Provide daily multiple vitamin	Provides vitamin requirements if nutrition is inadequate
Use soft brush or soft-tipped applicator for cleansing teeth; unwaxed dental floss	Prevents injury to oral cavity
Drink carbonated beverages, eat dry crackers in small amounts	Aids in controlling nausea
Provide listing of high protein and caloric, low fat foods that includes any food preferences and cultural restrictions	Assists in planning daily menus for optimal compliance

Discharge or Maintenance Evaluation

- Daily intake of 6 meals that include calculated caloric requirement and protein content

- Oral cavity free of redness, irritation, soreness or ulcerations after treatments (usually 4 weeks)
- Weight maintained within baseline determinations for height and frame
- Nausea and vomiting episodes decreased or absent
- Verbalized improved appetite and more interest in eating
- Able to develop menus that provide adequate nutritional intake
- Rests before and after meals; schedules meals around rest periods

Altered protection

Related to: Abnormal blood profiles (leukopenia, thrombocytopenia, anemia)
Defining characteristics: Deficient immunity, altered clotting, tissue hypoxia, weakness

Related to: Drug therapies (antineoplastic, corticosteroid)
Defining characteristics: Deficient immunity

Related to: Treatments (radiation for cancer)
Defining characteristics: Deficient immunity, weakness

Outcome Criteria

Reduced potential for infection, bleeding tendency, physical injury.

Interventions	Rationales
Assess presence of temperature elevation, chills, chest pain, decreased breath sounds with crackles, cough; foul-smelling cloudy urine with burning and frequency; redness, pain and drainage of skin or mucosa, breaks in pruritic areas	Bone marrow suppression caused by chemotherapy/radiation resulting in immunosuppression and abnormal blood profiles predisposes to infection in lungs, urinary tract, membranes of vagina, anus (leukopenia, anemia)

Interventions	Rationales
Assess skin for petechiae and ecchymosis, joint pain and swelling, blood in stool, urine, emesis	Immunosuppression causing thrombocytopenia as a result of chemotherapy/radiation; Hct and Hgb leads to anemia if bleeding is persistent
Assess presence of weakness, fatigue, activity tolerance	Results from anemia, anorexia, immobility caused by chemotherapy/radiation
Avoid invasive procedures when possible such as catheterization and injections	Prevents introduction of infectious agents and bleeding from trauma
Provide protective isolation if appropriate or avoid exposure to those with infections	Prevents exposure and transmission of organisms that may cause infection during immunosuppressed state
Use handwashing and sterile technique for care and procedures	Prevents exposure to potential infectious agents
Cleanse perianal area after bowel elimination with soft cloth or wipes	Promotes cleanliness and prevents tissue breakdown/infection
Cleanse female genitalia from front to back after urination and bowel elimination	Prevents urinary infection
Apply pressure to injection sites until bleeding stops	Prevents excessive bleeding
Maintain low position of bed, pad side rails, place articles within reach	Prevents trauma and falls
Assist in walking, offer aids to carry out ADL	Weakness and fatigue predisposes to falls

Information, Instruction, Demonstration

Interventions	Rationales
Avoid contact with those with infections	Reduces infection potential
Avoid blowing nose hard, straining at defecation; avoid aspirin	Increases potential for bleeding
Use electric razor, soft tooth brush or soft applicator to clean teeth and gums	Reduces potential for break in skin and bleeding
Maintain clear pathways, avoid rushing, use rails and other aids during activities	Reduces possibility of falls
Advise of importance of having blood test done as prescribed	Allows adjustments and evaluation of medications and potential for injury

Discharge or Maintenance Evaluation

- Patient can verbalize precautions to take to prevent infection, bleeding and falls
- Absence of pulmonary, urinary, skin, mucous membrane infections
- Bleeding episodes brought under control
- Absence of falls, trauma to skin, mucous membranes
- Fluid, nutritional intake maintained, rest and exercise pattern maintained
- Follow-up visits to physician and laboratory done as scheduled

Impaired skin integrity

Related to: External factor (radiation)
Defining characteristics: Destruction of skin layers, pruritus, skin discoloration

Related to: Internal factor (medications, altered metabolic state)
Defining characteristics: Diarrhea

Outcome Criteria

Skin intact and body image preserved.

Interventions	Rationales
Assess skin for rashes, itching, dryness, changes in color	Results from therapy regimen causing changes in sweat glands and destruction of epithelial cells
Assess anal and genitalia area for irritation, breakdown, amount and frequency of diarrhea	Results from rapid division of mucous membrane cells; diarrhea results from inflammation of gastrointestinal mucosa
Cleanse anal area after each bowel elimination with soft cloth or wipes	Prevents further damage
Apply A&D ointment or other protective cream	Decreased irritation and soreness caused by diarrhea
Wash skin using mild soap, warm water, gently pat dry; avoid washing or removing any radiation site marks	Prevents trauma to skin by harsh substances or treatment

Information, Instruction, Demonstration

Interventions	Rationales
Avoid scratching, sun exposure, use of tape, strong lotions, soaps, deodorants	Causes additional irritation to skin
Avoid use of hot or cold applications	Contraindicated when receiving radiation
Inform that vein discoloration and hyperpigmentation is temporary and clothing may cover areas	Preserves body image

Interventions	Rationales
Inform that nail ridges and thickening, failure to grow is temporary	Preserves body image

Discharge or Maintenance Evaluation

- Skin and muccous membranes intact
- Verbalizes statements reflecting changes caused by treatment regimen and ability to cope with temporary status of diarrhea, pruritis, alopecia
- Avoidance of substances harmful to skin to area

Body image disturbance

Related to: Biophysical factors (alopecia, colostomy, disfigurement of mastectomy)
Defining characteristics: Verbal response to actual change in structure and/or function, negative feelings about body/colostomy and mastectomy, physical change (alopecia) caused by chemotherapy, preoccupation with loss, change in social, physical involvement, persistent lymphedema of arm on affected side, inability to adjust to an alteration in sexual patterns

Outcome Criteria

Enhanced body image with adaptation to presence of colostomy and loss of breast and/or measures to conceal alopecia and restore body appearance.

Interventions	Rationales
Assess for responses to hair loss, presence of colostomy or mastectomy, effect on lifestyle and sexuality	Provides information about effect on body image and ability to adapt to and manage changes

Interventions	Rationales
Allow for expression of feelings about socializing and participating in activities; assure that a colostomy, prostatectomy, orchiectomy may affect sexual functioning but does not interfere with usual activities	Promotes venting of feelings and participation in social activities to prevent isolation, preserve sexual functioning

Information, Instruction, Demonstration

Interventions	Rationales
Inform of possible hair loss and return of hair growth after therapy with change in texture and color; also loss of beard, pubic hair, eyebrows and eyelashes	Result of chemotherapy
Suggest purchase of wig, scarf or hat if alopecia occurs; artificial eyelashes may also be purchased; purchase of well-fitting breast prosthesis	Hair loss may be uneven or complete and baldness may have a devastating effect on body image, similar effect on body image with loss of breast
Avoid use of rollers, dryers, hair spray, hard brush	Damages hair and promotes loss
Shampoo hair with mild soap and rinse well	Cleanses without damage to hair
Suggest ways to eliminate odor from colostomy drainage	Prevents embarrassing odors
Suggest loose and fully styled clothing	Conceals colostomy appliance
Inform to avoid sexual intercourse for 3-6 weeks following surgery	Permits tissue healing and prevents tissue trauma

Interventions	Rationales
Suggest sexual counseling or request information from physician	Provides information about alternative methods of sexual functioning
Initiate a visit from Reach To Recovery or Ostomy Club representative	Provides information and support from one who has undergone same or similar surgery
Suggest counseling for client and partner if appropriate	Provides support and assistance if adjustment difficulties present
Inform of mammoplasty procedures	Breast reconstruction enhances body image

Discharge or Maintenance Evaluation

- Verbalization of improved body image and progressive adaptation to colostomy, mastectomy
- Looks at colostomy, mastectomy
- Uses wig, clothing appropriate to change in body image, acquires breast prosthesis
- Participates in activities, resume friendships and relationships
- Participates in support groups, counseling as needed

Knowledge deficit

Related to: Lack of information about care of colostomy, prevention or treatment of lymphedema and care of remaining breast
Defining characteristics: Request for information, ability to care for colostomy, perform exercises to reduce edema on affected side and maintain shoulder mobility

Outcome Criteria

Appropriate care of colostomy; restoration of size and function of arm and shoulder on affected side.

Interventions	Rationales	Interventions	Rationales
Assist for knowledge of colostomy care and ability and desire to provide self-care of stoma and bowel elimination	Provides basis for instruction and demonstration of procedures necessary for self-care	Assess for knowledge and compliance in breast self-examination and mammography	Promotes early detection of abnormality in remaining breast
Use written instruction, visual aids in all instructions	Assists in effective teaching	Instruct to elevate affected arm on pillows, avoid any dependent position of arm; bed should be in semi-Fowler's position	Promotes drainage of fluid
Demonstrate setting up and administration of colostomy irrigation	Assists to establish regular pattern of elimination if colostomy is in descending colon	Encourage to flex and extend fingers early after surgery and increase arm and shoulder exercises daily	Prevents contractures and muscle shortening; maintains muscle tone and circulation
Instruct in cleansing of stoma and application of skin barrier or skin sealant and adhesive for appliance	Maintains cleanliness and prevents skin irritation from excreta	Refrain from using affected arm for BP monitoring	Constricts circulation and promotes swelling
Instruct in complete removal of appliance and materials with solvent, warm water and soap	Maintains skin integrity	Instruct in performance of hourly ROM exercises, progress from fingers to hand and wrist movements, then elbow flexion and extension hourly	Prevents contractures and promotes mobility of arm and shoulder
Instruct in measurement and appropriate application of appliance	Proper fit prevents leakage		
Demonstrate and instruct in emptying pouch including cleansing and reclosing with use of deodorant	Two-piece appliance allows for bag to be removed for emptying and only needs changing q 5 days	Continue instruction of post-mastectomy exercises by encouraging use of arm to brush hair, put on makeup, pulling rope attached to door knob, pulley over a shower rail, using fingers to climb up wall, flexion and extension of shoulder	Promotes lymph and blood circulation to prevent or control lymphedema and maintain use of arm and shoulder
Inform to avoid foods that are constipating gas forming, odor producing or irritating to the stoma	Promotes proper elimination via colostomy		
Instruct to report any change in color of stoma, diarrhea, constipation	Indication of disturbance in circulation to stoma	Inform to protect arm from trauma or sunburn; report any injury to physician	Infection common in arm that has circulatory problem
Assess for edema, pain and reduced movement in arm on affected side	Removal of lymph nodes impair lymph removal of fluid which results in edema	Inform of possible use of an elastic arm sleeve or intermittent pneumatic compression sleeve and device	Promotes circulation in arm in acute lymphedema by massage

Interventions	Rationales
Instruct and demonstrate BSE in remaining breast	Permits early detection of mass in breast by self-examination

Discharge or Maintenance Evaluation

- Performs care of colostomy stoma, peristomal skin, irrigation and appliance removal and application
- Avoids dietary intake that provokes colostomy dysfunction
- Requests assistance and/or asks questions when needed
- Performs BSE monthly, maintains health of remaining breast
- Lymphedema (chronic) maintained at minimal level
- Performs daily post-mastectomy exercises
- Arm and shoulder mobility on affected side returned and maintained
- Client verbalizes reasons why arm should be protected from trauma and carries out preventative measures
- Uses elastic arm sleeve during waking hours if prescribed with reduction in lymphedema

Breast Cancer

Genetic factors ↓

Hormonal factors ↓

Environmental factors ↓

External factors ↓

Mother, sister
with breast
cancer
↓

Increased
estrogen
↓

Chemicals
Radiation
Cigarette smoke
↓

Obesity
Diet
Virus
↓

Lump with malignant features (hard, irregular, fixed, painless)
Usually located in upper, outer part of breast
↓

Increased vascularity of breast
Skin edema and retraction
Axillary retraction
Axillary lymphadenopathy
↓

Infiltration, induration, dimpling of skin in later stage
↓

Metastasis to bone, lung, liver, brain

Colorectal Cancer

Aging   Familiar polyposis   Lack of dietary fiber   History of ulcerative colitis
↓   ↓   ↓   ↓

Colon mass, unknown factor
↓

Uncontrolled cell growth
↓

Invasion of mucosal and submucosal layer
↓

Invasion of entire wall of colon
↓

Invasion of serosal layer with regional lymph node involvement

↓   ↓

Metastasis   Bleeding from bowel
↓   Palpated mass
           Change in bowel habits (constipation/diarrhea)
Liver   Bowel obstruction
Lungs   Pain (late symptom)
Bone
Lymphatic system

Leukemia

Genetic factor   Acquired disease   Chemical and physical agents

↓   ↓   ↓

Transformation of lymphocytes or granulocytes

↓   ↓

Chronic lymphocytic leukemia   Chronic granulocytic leukemia

↓   ↓

Abnormal mature WBC in peripheral circulation
Diffuse replacement of bone marrow with leukemic cells

↓

Infiltration of liver, spleen, lymph nodes and other body tissues
Infection in any organ

↓

Fever, chills, night sweats
Weakness, fatigue (anemia)
Bleeding of skin and mucous membranes (thrombocytopenia)
Weight loss (hypermetabolism of leukemic cells)
Headache, visual disturbances (CNS involvement)
Abdominal tenderness and fullness (hepatomegaly, splenomegaly, lymphadomegaly)

Lung Cancer

Smoking	Environmental hazards: air pollution, asbestos, chemicals	Metastasis from a primary site	Age
↓	↓	↓	↓

← Reduced efficiency of immune system

↓

Bronchogenic carcinoma

↓	↓	↓	↓
Epidermoid or Squamous cell	Large cell	Adenocarcinoma	Small cell (oat)
↓	↓	↓	↓
Arises from basal reserve cells		Arises from mucin-secreting cells	Arises from K-type cells
↓	↓	↓	↓
Central lung location	Lung periphery location		Hilar location
→	↓		←

Bronchial irritation and obstruction	Mediastinum invasion	Pleural space invasion	Blood vessel invasion
↓	↓	↓	↓
Cough Dyspnea Rhonchi	Dull, intermittent pain Hoarseness Dysphagia	Persistent, severe pain Dyspnea Pleural effsion Atelectasis	Hemoptysis Decreased venous driamage from head, neck, chest wall
↓	↓	↓	↓

Metastasis to bone, brain, liver, lymph nodes

Prostate Cancer

Aging   Endocrine factors
↓   ↓

Adenocarcinoma in posterior liobe of prostate
↓

Extension of tumor beyond capsule of prostate
Metastatic infiltration

↓   ↓

Pelvis lymph nodes   Difficulty starting or stopping urination
Bone   Dysuria
Lungs   Frequency
Liver   Hematuria
                                    Hard, enlarged, fixed prostate

Transition to Home/Long-Term Facility

Older adult

↓

Unable to manage self-care	Loss of independence	Prior hospitalization
Chronic debilitating illness	and autonomy	

↓ (left) ↓ (center) ↓ (right)

Voluntary placement
Involuntary placement
Family involvement and needs

↓

Need for personal territory
Need to be included in decision
Emotional preparation

↓

Preadmission planning
Discharge planning

↓ (left)   ↓ (center)   ↓ (right)

Maldajustment   Adjustment

↓   ↓

Anger   Disorganization
Abandonment   Reorganization
Depression   Relationship building
Insensitive family judgments,   Stabilization
   guilt, conflicts
Loss of self-esteem

Transition to Home/Long-Term Facility

Under normal conditions, the older adult lives in a home or apartment type dwelling that allows for autonomy and privacy. Leaving this environment with all familiar belongings and memories to live with family members or in a long-term facility creates a sense of loss for the individual. Adjustment to relocation depends on minimal trauma during transition accomplished by proper emotional preparation, participation in the admission planning and decision-making process, and family acceptance.

NURSING CARE PLANS

Essential nursing diagnoses and plans associated with this condition

Altered thought process (70)

Related to: Psychological conflicts, physiological changes
Defining characteristics: Impaired ability for self-care, altered sleep pattern, anxiety, feeling of abandonment, presence of family conflict, involuntary placement or relocation

SPECIFIC DIAGNOSIS AND CARE PLANS

Relocation stress syndrome

Related to: Decreased physical health status, lack of support system, feeling of powerlessness, past, concurrent, and recent losses, moderate to high degree of environmental change
Defining characteristics: Change in environment/location, increased confusion, anxiety and apprehension, insecurity, sad affect, withdrawal, vigilance, verbalization of unwillingness to relocate or transfer

Outcome Criteria

Phases of relocation adjustment achieved with adaptation to new environment

Interventions	Rationales
Assess the need for new living quarters, feelings about loss of personal possessions, loneliness, meaning of independence and feelings about sudden dependence	Provides information useful in assisting adaptation to the new environment
Assess for anxiety, anger, depression, and other negative emotions	Responses to trauma or relocation
Familiarize with admission process and planning; allow to participate in decisions regarding daily needs	Promotes smooth transition and some control over the environment
Discuss feelings of family during relocations and presence of guilt, conflict and/or supporting behaviors	Family attitude can interfere with and create problems with adjustment

Interventions	Rationales
Provide privacy and personal space, personal objects; allow to arrange items and furniture in own room	Promotes satisfaction with new environment

Information, Instruction, Demonstration

Interventions	Rationales
Encourage familiar coping skills, anxiety reduction techniques	Increases autonomy and improves self-esteem
Inform of choices to make regarding daily care and leisure activities within physical and mental limitations	Promotes independence and empowers client to meet obligations and responsibilities
Review discharge plan and discuss implementation with client and family	Provides continuity of care if discharged from a hospital

Discharge or Maintenance Evaluation

- Progressive movement through phases of adjustment
- Maintains autonomy, privacy, and personal space
- Manages self-care and choice of activities within identified limitations
- Participates in decision-making regarding planning of daily routines

Appendix

Appendix

ANA STANDARDS OF GERONTOLOGICAL NURSING PRACTICE

Standard I

Data are systematically and continuously collected about the health status of the older adult. The data are accessible, communicated, and recorded

Standard II

Nursing diagnoses are derived from the identified normal responses of the individual to aging and the data collected about the health status of the older adult

Standard III

A plan of nursing care is developed in conjunction with the older adult and/or significant other(s) that includes goals derived from the nursing diagnosis

Standard IV

The plan of nursing care includes priorities and prescribed nursing approaches and measures to achieve the goals derived from the nursing diagnosis

Standard V

The plan of care is implemented, using appropriate nursing actions

Standard VI

The older adult and/or significant other(s) participate in determining the progress attained in the achievement of established goals

Standard VII

The older adult and/or significant other(s) participate in the ongoing process of assessment, the setting of new goals, the recording of priorities, the revision of plan for nursing care, and the initiation of new nursing action

INDEX OF NURSING DIAGNOSES (NANDA)*

Activity intolerance

Activity intolerance, risk for

Adaptive capacity, decreased: intracranial

Adjustment, impaired

Airway clearance, ineffective

Anxiety

Aspiration, risk for

Body image disturbance

Body temperature, altered, risk for

Bowel incontinence

Breastfeeding, effective

Breastfeeding, ineffective

Breastfeeding, interrupted

Breathing pattern, ineffective

Cardiac ouptut, decreased

Caregiver role strain

Caregiver role strain, risk for

Communication, impaired verbal

Community coping, potential for enhanced

Community coping, ineffective

Confusion, acute

Confusion, chronic

Constipation

Constipation, colonic

Constipation, perceived

Coping, defensive

Coping, family: potential for growth

Coping, ineffective family: compromised

Coping, ineffective family: disabling

Coping, ineffective individual

Decisional conflict (specify)

Denial, ineffective

Diarrhea

Disuse syndrome, risk for

Diversional activity deficit

Dysreflexia

Energy field disturbance

Environmental interpretation syndrome: impaired

Family processes, altered: alcoholism

Family processes, altered

Fatigue

Fear

Fluid volume deficit

Fluid volume deficit, risk for

Fluid volume excess

Gas exchange, impaired

Grieving, anticipatory

Grieving, dysfunctional

Growth and development, altered

Health maintenance, altered

Health-seeking behaviors (specify)

Home maintenance management, impaired

Hopelessness

Hyperthermia

Hypothermia

Incontinence, functional

Incontinence, reflex

*Derived from revised 1994 Eleventh Conference of Official Nursing Diagnoses presnted by the North American Nursing Diagnosis Association (NANDA).

Incontinence, stress

Incontinence, total

Incontinence, urge

Infant behavior, disorganized

Infant behavior, disorganized: risk for

Infant behavior, organized: potential for enhanced

Infant feeding pattern, ineffective

Infection, risk for

Injury, perioperative positioning, risk for

Injury, risk for

Knowledge deficit (specify)

Loneliness, risk for

Management of therapeutic regimen, community: ineffective

Management of therapeutic regimen, families: ineffective

Management of therapeutic regimen, individuals: effective

Management of therapeutic regimen, individuals: ineffective

Memory, impaired

Mobility, impaired physical

Noncompliance (specify)

Nutrition, altered: less than body requirements

Nutrition, altered: more than body requirements

Nutrition, altered: risk for more than body requirements

Oral mucous membrane, altered

Pain

Pain, chronic

Parent/Infant/Child attachment altered, risk for

Parental role conflict

Parenting, altered

Parenting, altered, risk for

Peripheral neurovascular dysfunction, risk for

Personal identity disturbance

Poisoning, risk for

Post-trauma response

Powerlessness

Protection, altered

Rape-trauma syndrome

Rape-trauma syndrome: compound reaction

Rape-trauma syndrome: silent reaction

Relocation stress syndrome

Role performance, altered

Self-care deficit, bathing/hygiene

Self-care deficit, dressing/grooming

Self-care deficit, feeding

Self-care deficit, toileting

Self-esteem disturbance

Self-esteem, chronic low

Self-esteem, situational low

Self-mutilation, risk for

Sensory/perceptual alterations (specify) (visual, auditory, kinesthetic, gustatory, tactile, olfactory)

Sexual dysfunction

Sexuality patterns, altered

Skin integrity, impaired

Skin integrity, impaired, risk for

Sleep pattern disturbance

Social interaction, impaired

Social isolation

Spiritual distress (distress of the human spirit)

Spiritual well-being, potential for enhanced

Suffocation, risk for

Swallowing, impaired

Thermoregulation, ineffective

Thought processes, altered

Tissue integrity, impaired

Tissue perfusion, altered (specify type) (renal, cerebral, cardiopulmonary, gastrointestinal, peripheral)

Trauma, risk for

Unilateral neglect

Urinary elimination, altered

Urinary retention

Ventilation, inability to sustain spontaneous

Ventilatory weaning process, dysfunctional

Violence, risk for: self-directed or directed at others

ABBREVIATIONS

ADL	Activities of daily living
BP	Blood pressure
CAD	Coronary artery disease
Cl	Chloride
CVA	Cerebrovascular accident
ECG	Electrocardiogram
g	Gram
Hct	Hematocrit
Hb	Hemoglobin
hr	Hour
IM	Intramuscular
I&O	Intake and output
IV	Intravenous
K	Potassium
L	Liter
LOC	Level of conscience
MI	Myocardial infarction
mg	Milligram
min	Minute
mL	Mililiter
Na	Sodium
P	Phosphorus
PO	Orally
REM	Rapid eye movement
SC	Subcutaneous
SL	Sublingual
TIA	Transient ischemic attack
VS	Vital signs

ASSESSMENT SCALES AND TOOLS FOR ANALYSIS OF MENTAL/SOCIAL/ PHYSICAL STATUS IN THE OLDER ADULT

Older American Research and Service Center Instrument (OARS)
    Focus is multidimensional assessment of functional abilities in social, economic resources; mental and physical health; activities of daily living (ADL)

Norton Scale
    Focus is to measure the risk for development of pressure sores based on assessment of five areas (mental and physical condition, activity and mobility, and incontinence) with four levels associated with each area assessed

Braden Scale
    Focus is on skin assessment to predict risk for pressure sores that includes six areas (activity, mobility, nutrition, sensory perception, moisture, friction, shearing) with four degrees of limitations in each area

Katz Index of ADL
    Focus is to assess level of independence in activities of daily living (bathing, grooming, dressing, toileting, feeding, ambulation, tranferring, continence)

Tinetti Gait and Balance Scale
    Focus is to assess the risk of falls in the older adult with evaluation of balance and gait by observation of specific maneuvers while sitting, standing, and walking

Family APGAR
    Focus is to screen social functioning of the older adult by assessment of specific categories (affection, growth, partnership, adaptation, and resolve)

Social Competence Activities
    Focus is on assessment of changes in ability to perform activities in the home, work, recreational and social activities

Music Therapy Assessment Tool
    Focus is on evaluation of music therapy in those with Alzheimer's Disease

Glasgow Coma Scale (GCS)
    Focus is to evaluate level of consciousness with orientation, verbal and motor responses

SET Test
    Focus is to assess dementia by demonstrating ability to identify a set of ten items (fruits, colors, animals, towns)

Haycox Dementia Behavior Scale
    Focus is on assessment of behaviors indicating varied degrees of dementia

Dementia Mood Assessment
    Focus is on the assessment of mood and behavior

Short Portable Mental Status Questionnaire (SPMSQ)
    Focus is on cognitive and affective assessment to determine intellectual impairment by the use of ten questions that test orientation, memory, and mathematical ability

Global Deterioration Scale (GDS)
    Focus is on age-related cognitive decline and Alzheimer's Disease by assessment of stage of decline based on clinical characteristics associated with forgetfulness, followed by levels of confusion and dementia

Functional Assessment Stages (FAST)
    Focus is on assessment of normal aging and Alzheimer's Disease by evaluating cognitive deterioration associated with confusion and dementia

Mini-Mental State Exam (MMSE)
    Focus is on assessment of cognitive function (orientation, attention and calculation, language, recall, and registration)

Beck Depression Inventory

Focus is to assess the severity of depression by evaluating thirteen items that are associated with symptoms and attitudes of depression

Hamilton Rating Scale for Depression (Ham-D)

Focus is an inventory of items to assess depression

Yesavage Geriatric Depression Scale

Focus is to screen for mood and behavior associated with possible depression

Zung Self-Rating Depression Scale (SDS)

Focus is to assess level of depression

Inventory of Psychic and Somatic Complaints of the Elderly (IPSCE)

Focus is to assess somatic manifestations of psychologic conditions

Minnesota Multiphasic Personality Inventory

Focus is on lengthly questionnaire to assess for potential personality disorders

Geriatric Hopelessness Scale

Focus is on assessment of subclinical depression in the older adult and level of hopelessness

MEDICATION CONSIDERATIONS FOR THE OLDER ADULT

Medication regimens for most elderly commonly include single or multiple drugs prescribed for one or more conditions. Drugs must be evaluated singly and in combination with other drugs for adverse effects, drug-drug interactions, drug-food interactions, and pharmacokinetic, pharmacodynamic, psychodynamic considerations associated with possible general physical and mental changes related to the aging process.

1. **Pharmacokinetics:**

   Absorption:
   Reduced blood flow to the gastrointestinal organs can decrease absorption

   Reduced motility can increase the amount of the drug absorbed

   Reduced gastric acid can decrease absorption if a low pH is required for some drugs

   Distribution:
   Increased adipose and decreased muscle mass and water content can allow more to be distributed and affect the half-life

   Increased adipose allows for drugs that are stored in this tissue to accumulate and remain in the body longer

   Decreased water volume can reduce volume distribution of water-soluble drugs and increased volume distribution of fat-soluble drugs

   Decreased serum albumin can increase blood level of a drug and cause toxicity and protein-bound drugs administered together can compete for protein molecules leaving a reduced effect of those drugs that do not bind effectively

   Metabolism:
   Hepatic changes can increase drug levels leading to prolonged action of the drug

   Cigarette smoking can increase metabolism of drugs by its effect on liver enzymes and create a need for higher dosage

   Excretion:
   Reduced number of nephrons, renal filtration, and blood flow can increase the time needed to eliminate drugs and cause an increase in the elimination half-life resulting in toxicity or paradoxical effects

2. **Pharmacodynamics:**

   Routes of administration:
   Choice based on the known biologic and therapeutic effect of the drug at the proposed site of action or organ; can be oral (PO), intramuscular (IM), intravenous (IV), subcutaneous (SC), topical (TOP), rectal (RECT), vaginal (VAG), eye (OPHTH), ear (OTO), inhalation (INH)

   As muscle mass decreases, so do sites appropriate for injections of medications

   Drug action times:
   Onset of action, peak effect, duration of action

3. **Psychodynamics:**
   Confusion, decreased visual acuity can result in misreading of labels, leading to repeated doses or forgetting to take the drugs (overdose or reduced effect), especially in regimens involving multiple medications and doses

   Confusion states can be caused by psychotropics, sedatives/hypnotics, and narcotic analgesics

   Decreased elimination of drugs can manifest altered thought processes leading to overdosage and toxicity

   Chemical restraint is not considered an option for the older adult population

4. **Drug Administration:**

Self-administration of medication regimen depends on dexterity, memory, judgement, auditory or visual acuity, complete knowledge of drugs, and if drug abuse a possibility

Assess misuse of over-the-counter drugs (laxatives, analgesics, sleep medications); these should be avoided unless advised by physician to avoid interactions with prescribed drugs

Select oral drug forms on an individual basis as available (liquid, chewable, sprinkles or powders, tablet that can be crushed or dissolved) or sustained release and enteric coated tablets or capsules

Use of reminders to take medications (alarm clock, daily check-off list, con-tainer with labeled compartments)

Note names of more than one physician on prescription drugs and investigate if each knows what the other is prescribing

Divide dosage regimens if behaviors are drug-related (mood changes) or consider possible drug holiday in long-term use of a drug to reduce risk of accumulation of drug or toxicity

Review drug regimen for drug-drug or drug-food interactions, possible decreased fluid intake that can result in inappropriate drug interactions

Adjust or decrease dosage if prolonged action is suspected or signs and symptoms noted, or in long-term regimens if side effects and change in effectiveness warrants this

Administer medications as prescribed with precautions to ensure safety and effective results; evaluate for desired effects, untoward effects, and of any new medications added to the regimen Ensure compliance with all periodic laboratory testing associated with drug levels or effects on other body systems depending on medication regimen

5. **Drug Misuse/Abuse:**

The use of medications for a reason not indicated by a particular drug is con-sidered misuse

The inappropriate use of drugs that disrupt functioning and relationships leading to psychological dependence is considered abuse

Misuse and abuse of substances include prescribed and over-the-counter medications, nicotine (smoking), caffeine (coffee, tea, chocolate)

Most abused drug in the older population is alcohol

Common causes for substance abuse are chronic illness, loneliness, retirement and disengagement, loss of loved ones, friends and relationships, financial security, and personal belongings

SELECTED NATIONAL AGENCIES

Administration on Aging
Department of Health and Human Services
330 Independence Ave., S.W.
Washington, D.C. 20201

National Council on the Aging
600 Maryland Ave., S.W.
West Wing 100
Washington, D.C. 20024

American Geriatrics Society
770 Lexington Ave., Suite 300
New York, NY 10021

American Nurses' Association
Council on Gerontological Nursing Practice
600 Maryland Ave. SW, Suite 100W
Washington, DC 20024

Gerontological Society of America
1275 K St, NW, Suite 350
Washington, DC 20005

American Association for Geriatric Psychiatry
PO Box 376-A
Greenbelt, MD 20768

Nursing Home Information Service Center
1331 F St, Suite 500
Washington, DC 20004

American Association of Retired Persons
1909 K St. NW
Washington, DC 20049

American Dietetic Association
216 W Jackson Blvd, Suite 800
Chicago, IL 60606

American Heart Association
7320 Greenville Ave.
Dallas, TX 75231

American Lung Association
1740 Broadway
New York, NY 10019

American Cancer Society
777 Third Ave.
New York, NY 10017

American Diabetes Association
149 Madison Ave.
New York, NY 10016

United Ostomy Association
2001 W Beverly Blvd.
Los Angeles, CA 90057

Help for Incontinent People
Box 544
Union, SC 29389

Emphysema Anonymous
PO Box 66
Fort Myers, FL 33902

Arthritis Foundation
3400 Peachtree Rd., Suite 1101
Atlanta, GA 30326

American Parkinson's Disease Association
116 John St.
New York, NY 10038

National Multiple Sclerosis Society
733 Third Ave.
New York, NY 10017

Mental Health Association
1800 N Kent St.
Arlington, VA 22209

Association for Alzheimer's Disease and Related Disorders
919 N Michigan Ave., Suite 1000
Chicago, IL 60611

American Council of the Blind
1156 15 St, NW, Suite 720
Washington, DC 20005

National Association for the Deaf
814 Thayer Ave.
Silver Spring, MD 20910

National Kidney Foundation
1 Park Ave.
New York, NY 10016

SELECTED PUBLICATIONS

Aging
Department of Health and Human Services
200 Independence Ave, SW
Washington, DC 20201

Journal of the American Geriatrics Society
Williams and Wilkins Co
428 E Preston St
Baltimore, MD 21202

Long-Term Care Currents
Ross Laboratories
625 Cleveland Ave
Columbus, OH 43216

The Gerontologist
Gerontological Society of America
1275 K ST, NW, Suite 350
Washington, DC 200005

Modern Maturity
American Association of Retired Persons
3200 E Carson St
Lakewood, CA 90712

REFERENCES

Abrams, WB and Berkow, R (Ed): *The Merck Manual of Geriatrics*, Rahway, NJ, Merck Sharp and Dohme Research Laboratories, 1990.

American Nurses' Association: *Standards and Scope of Gerontological Nursing Practice*, Kansas City, 1987.

Beckingham, AC: *Promoting Healthy Aging: A Nursing and Community Perspective*, St. Louis, Mosby Year Book, 1993.

Black, JM and Matassarin-Jacobs: *Luckmann and Sorensen's Medical-Surgical Nursing: A Psychophysiologic Approach*, ed 4, Philadelphia, WB Saunders, 1993.

Burke, MM and Walsh, MB: *Gerontological Nursing: Care of the Frail Elderly*, St. Louis, Mosby Year Book, 1992.

Burnside, IM: *Nursing and the Aged*, ed 3, New York, McGraw-Hill, 1988.

Butler, RN, Lewis, M, and Sunderland, T: *Aging and Mental Health*, ed 4, New York, Macmillan, 1991.

Calkins, E, Ford, AB, and Katz, PR (Eds): *Practice of Geriatrics*, ed 2, Philadelphia, WB Saunders, 1992.

Carpenito, LJ: *Nursing Diagnosis: Application to Clinical Practice*, Philadelphia Lippincott, 1992.

Chenitz, WC, Stone, JT, and Salisbury, SA (Eds): *Clinical Gerontological Nursing*, Philadelphia, WB Saunders, 1991.

Christiansen, JL and Grzybowski, JM: *Biology of Aging*, St. Louis, Mosby Year Book, 1993.

Eliopoulos, C: *Legal Risks in the Long-Term Care Facility*, Glen Arm, MD, Health Education Network, 1991.

Eliopoulos, C: *Manual of Gerontologic Nursing*, St. Louis, Mosby Year Book, 1995.

Ferri, RS: *Care Planning for the Older Adult: Nursing Diagnosis in Long-Term Care*, Philadelphia, WB Saunders, 1994.

Fowles, D (Ed): *A Profile of Older Americans*, Washington DC, American Association of Retired Persons, 1993.

Gettrust, KV and Brabec, PD: *Nursing Diagnosis in Clinical Practice: Guides for Care Planning*, Albany, Delmar, 1992.

Hamdy, RC, et al: *Alzheimer's Disease: A Handbook for Caregivers*, ed 2, St. Louis, Mosby Year Book, 1994.

Heckheimer, EF: *Health Promotion of the Elderly in the Community*, Philadelphia, WB Saunders, 1989.

Hogstel, MO (Ed): *Clinical Manual of Gerontological Nursing*, St. Louis, Mosby Year Book, 1992.

Hogstel, MO: *Geropsychiatric Nursing*, ed 2, St. Louis, Mosby Year Book, 1995.

Hogstel, MO (Ed): *Nursing Care of the Older Adult*, ed 3, Albany, Delmar, 1994.

Johnson-Pawlson, J: *Quest for Quality*, Washington DC, American Health Care Association, 1991.

Katz, BR: *Geriatric Pharmacology*, New York, McGraw-Hill, 1993.

Lewis, SM and Collier, IC: *Medical-Surgical Nursing: Assessment and Management of Clinical Problems*, ed 3, St. Louis, Mosby Year Book, 1992.

Loftis, PA and Glover, T: *Decision Making in Gerontologic Nursing*, St. Louis, Mosby Year Book, 1993.

Lueckenote, AG: *Pocket Guide to Gerontologic Assessment*, ed 2, St. Louis, Mosby Year Book, 1994.

Maas, M, Buckwalter, K, and Hardy, M: *Nursing Diagnosis and New Interventions for the Elderly*, Redwood City, CA, Addison-Wesley, 1991.

Matteson, MA and McConnell, ES: *Gerontological Nursing: Concepts and Practice*, Philadelphia, WB Saunders, 1988.

McCloskey, JC and Bulechek, GM: *Nursing Interventions Classification (NIC)*, St. Louis, Mosby Year Book, 1992.

North American Nursing Diagnosis Association, *Official Nursing Diagnoses of the Eleventh Conference*, St. Louis, 1994-1995.

Rogers-Seidl, FF (Ed): *Geriatric Nursing Care Plans*, St. Louis, Mosby Year Book, 1991.

Salzman, C (Ed): *Clinical Geriatric Psychopharmacology*, ed 2, Baltimore, Williams and Williams, 1992.

Skidmore-Roth, L: *Nursing Drug Reference*, St. Louis, Mosby Year Book, 1995.

Sodeman, WA: *Instructions for Geriatric Patients*, Philadelphia, WB Saunders, 1995.

Stanley, M and Beare, PG (Eds): *Gerontological Nursing*, Philadelphia, FA Davis, 1995.

Watson, J and Jaffe, MS: *Nurse's Manual of Laboratory and Diagnostic Tests*, ed 2, Philadelphia, FA Davis, 1995.

Weiner, M (Ed): *The Dementias: Diagnosis and Management*, Washington DC, American Psychiatric Press, 1991.

Wolf, RS and Pellemer, KA: *Helping Elderly Victims: The Reality of Elder Abuse*, New York, Columbia University Press, 1989.

Order Form

____ Handbook of Long Term Care $18.00

____ Nurse Assistant Handbook $17.00

____ The Nurse's Survival Guide $29.95

____ The Body in Brief $29.95

____ The Nurse's Trivia Calendar $9.95

____ Diagnostic and Laboratory Cards $24.95

____ Procedure Cards for Clinical Use $21.95

____ Geriatric Nutrition and Diet Therapy (2nd ed.) $17.95

____ Pediatric Nursing Care Plans $31.95

____ RN NCLEX Review Cards $26.95

____ PN/VN Review Cards $26.95

____ Geratric Nursing Care Plans (2nd ed.) $31.95

____ Geratric Outline $22.95

____ Infection Control $84.00

____ Quality Assurance in Long-Term Care $62.95

Name

Address

City, State, Zip

Phone: (   )

☐ Visa   ☐ Mastercard   ☐ American Express   ☐ Check/Money Order Attached

Card No.

Expiration Date:

Signature:

**Prices Subject to Change.
Please add $4.00 each for postage and handling.
Include your local sales tax.**

Skidmore-Roth Publishing, Inc.

**2620 S. Parker Road, #147
Aurora, Colorado 80014**

1-800-825-3150